It's me again, doctor

Andrew Hamilton was born in Scotland and grew up in Kent. He studied medicine at Cambridge University and King's College Hospital, London. At Cambridge, he gained a blue for rugby and a half-blue as a heavyweight boxer. He was also capped ten times by Scotland at rugby. Shortly after qualifying as a doctor, he left England for Kenya, where he worked for eight years at a mission hospital. Returning home because of ill-health in the family, he settled into general practice.

It's me again, doctor is his second collection of stories giving delightful insights into the pathos and humour of his medical work and family life, a sequel to his bestselling *Sorry to bother you, doctor*. His easy yet perceptive style amuses and entertains. And his encounters with patients often result in more than just an improvement in their health . . .

Andrew Hamilton is now retired, and wonders how he ever found time to be a doctor. His interests include gardening, bird-watching and fishing, the life of his local church, and teaching his grandchildren how to handle a rugger ball.

'Andrew Hamilton' is a pseudonym.

IT'S ME AGAIN DOCTOR

ANDREW HAMILTON

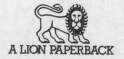

A LION PAPERBACK

Copyright © 1983 Andrew Hamilton

Published by
Lion Publishing plc
Icknield Way, Tring, Herts, England
ISBN 0 85648 575 6
Lion Publishing Corporation
10885 Textile Road, Ypsilanti, Michigan 48197, USA
ISBN 0 85648 575 6
Albatross Books
PO Box 320, Sutherland, NSW 2232, Australia
ISBN 0 86760 447 6

First edition 1983

Author's note
The stories in this book are mostly drawn from real
life; however, to preserve the anonymity of those
involved, not all details are accurate, and the names
of some people and places have been altered.

British Library Cataloguing in Publication Data

Hamilton, Andrew, 1916–
   It's me again doctor.
   1. Family medicine—Great Britain—Anecdotes,
   facetiae, satire, etc.
   I. Title
   362.1'72'0942   R729.G4

   ISBN 0–85648–575–6

Printed and bound in Great Britain
by Collins, Glasgow

Contents

She sat there, her arm resting easily on my desk, blue eyes dancing with the pleasure of reminiscence.

'Odd, isn't it, doctor, my 'Rene being older than my brother Keith an' he hasn't even got a regular girl-friend yet? And 'Rene getting married next week an' all.'

My patient herself was a happy exception to a general rule. Married at sixteen, she had a steady husband, three nice kids, and they were saving to buy their own house.

She laughed again. 'Coo! I remember you comin' to Mum that night. I guess it was the midwife called you out when she found Keith had his cord twisted twice round his neck. Got it off all right, you did – you must've done, mustn't you, seein' he's here now. Saw you comin' down the stairs after, remember? Jimmy and me had the back bedroom with 'Rene in a cot between us. Proper houseful we were, I can tell you. As for you – hadn't even stopped to comb your hair before comin', and there you were with your pyjama-cord hanging out of the top of your trousers! You didn't 'alf look a sight, doctor! Laugh, I couldn't help myself, even though poor old Mum had been goin' through it upstairs.'

I remembered that the baby had had fine auburn hair, not unlike that of his sister sitting there.

She got up, took the prescription I was holding out, smiled again. 'Ta, doctor,' she said, and went out.

The visit from this friendly girl with ginger hair and her recollection of her brother Keith's delivery set me thinking. It was eighteen years since I had begun in the practice, and a lot had happened in those eighteen years – in the world at large, and in our sleepy south coast home-

7

town of Wilverton. I allowed myself the luxury of a little reminiscing too.

I recalled the holiday when my wife, Elisabeth, and I and Sarah, our daughter, had stopped for the night at a 'Bed and Breakfast (with evening meal) Terms Reasonable' in a Cotswold village near Bourton-on-the-Water. Before our 'meal', I went for a stroll down the hill to develop an appetite after sitting all day in the car.

At the bottom I found an ancient stone bridge crossing a stream. I approached stealthily and looked cautiously over the parapet. Clear limestone water fell into a little pool in a cascade.

Yes! As I guessed, there was a brown trout: he was about three-quarters of a pound in weight, and he was lying, tail waving slowly, in an eddy. As I watched, he suddenly swirled forward to take a trifle which came down the cascade from under the bridge, then curved gracefully back to his lie.

I watched fascinated as this little performance was re-enacted three or four times and then went away, cheered and ready for my supper. . .

Sitting in the surgery, it now seemed to me that the 'water under the bridge' was running clear again and my mind was busy snapping up the morsels that came through on the current. Eighteen years as a general practitioner had certainly provided a whole variety of experiences – some good, some bad.

'I must write them all down,' I decided, 'before they become absorbed and forgotten again. But I mustn't discard the bad, as the trout occasionally did. That would hardly be honest.'

1
The west wind

I walked up the path, humming. 'Summer suns are glowing over land and sea' is not a hymn I like especially, but it just seemed to fit the day. There was a brass ring hanging from a lion's mouth, fastened to the door. I gave it three sharp knocks and waited.

There was a few seconds' pause before I saw, through the stained-glass panels, a figure approaching: short – five feet four at the most. Strange, I thought; with a name like 'Edward Gascoigne', the man I was expecting should have been tall, impressive, probably with black eyebrows and a hawk-nose – an altogether commanding presence.

The Yale lock clicked back and a wispy-haired little man with drooping moustache peered out. 'Yes?' His eyes lighted on my bag. 'Oh, coom ter see the missus, 'aven't yer?' His accent suggested a concentration of Cockney with just a hint of Sussex.

'Yes, I'm Doctor Hamilton,' I answered. 'I was asked to come and see your wife.'

He held out his left hand to me in greeting. I changed my bag over to the right and shook it. He caught my eyes examining his right hand. It was contracted like a claw and the two middle fingers were missing. 'Stopped a bit of Jerry shell-case in the '14–'18, doctor. Lucky not to lose me 'ole bloomin' 'and.'

He shut the door. It was difficult to see in the dark little hall-way after the brightness of the sunshine outside, but I made out the staircase beyond the umbrella-stand. 'Lead the way, would you?' I pointed upstairs.

'Nah, doctor, she's in the front, dahn 'ere.' He opened the door on his left. 'Nellie.' His voice was soft and gentle. ''ere's the doctor come ter see yer, Nellie. Coom by, doctor.'

He stood back and I went into the sunlit front room. It was half-filled by a double iron bedstead with brass knobs. More than half-filling the bed, in a sort of recumbent regality, lay a lady who would have made two of Edward Gascoigne without the least difficulty. Beautiful, snow-white, wavy hair framed a charming, chubby countenance. The ample bosom rose and fell with great rapidity beneath a nightie besprinkled with pink roses.

'This 'ere's Doctor Hamilton, Nellie. Nice of 'im to coom so quick, in't it?'

Nellie smiled a brief little smile, but her expression was really one of mute appeal. She was breathing rapidly, but her pink cheeks suggested panic rather than lack of oxygen.

I nodded to her and smiled back, put my bag on the foot of her bed and took her wrist. Her pulse was regular but almost uncountable. I sat down beside her.

'Now, what do you feel's the trouble?'

'Doctor, it's these attacks. This one started this morning. It's a sort of fluttering here.' With a queenly gesture, she laid her podgy fingers over her left breast. 'I come all over swimey and I can't get my breath.' While she was distracted talking, her breathing had become normal.

'Now I want you to breathe slowly and quietly,' I said. 'You will feel better.'

I did a quick examination of her – heart, lungs and blood pressure. I would have been glad of an electrocardiogram – but even without it the diagnosis was clear. She hadn't been so far out with her 'fluttering': she was suffering from a paroxysm of 'auricular flutter' – a sudden racing of the beats of the small chambers of the heart, but with only a proportion of them getting through to the ventricles, the large chambers. At her age, this was almost certainly due to hardened arteries. It wasn't immediately dangerous, but the sooner we could stop it, the better. Sometimes a trick manoeuvre would do it. I decided to try.

'Now, Mrs Gascoigne, I'm going to do something which isn't very comfortable but it may help you. Just close your eyes.'

I pressed both closed eyes with a thumb and forefinger,

and with the other thumb massaged a carotid artery. She shrank away a little – understandable considering the size of my digits – then she cried out, 'Doctor, I feel better!'

I released the pressure, picked up my stethoscope and listened to her heart. It was still going too fast but was not far off normal now. Her china-blue eyes had lost their panic and she looked at me with something akin to reverence.

I turned to Edward. He was grinning (even his moustache looked more jaunty), and he was giving the thumbs-up sign with his good hand.

'Would you get down to the chemist and have this made up?' I wrote out a prescription for Digoxin, the active principle of the foxglove leaf, and for Quinidine, a near-relative of quinine. Together they would stabilize her heart.

'I'll come and see you tomorrow, but you can get up and sit in the window.' Over the country road the fields lay warm in the sunshine. That view should tempt her, I thought. Nellie, however, displayed no enthusiasm for leaving her brass-bound throne.

Next day her heart-rate had improved and was almost normal, but there she was still in bed, securely ensconced and obviously content.

'Now, Nellie . . .' My familiarity made her blush a deeper shade of pink. 'When I come tomorrow, I want you *up*! It's not good for you to remain inactive too long, so – you have been warned.'

In the little hall, Edward put a finger to his lips and beckoned me. We went into their tiny back kitchen.

''Scuse me bringing you in 'ere, doctor, but can I 'ave a word in your ear? Now Nellie – she's not lazy, it's just she's got used to me doin' things for 'er. We git on like an 'ouse on fire, never no cross words. Fact, it's our golden wedding in three months' time. So go easy on 'er, doctor, wouldn't want her upset.'

'Look, Edward, it's only for her own good. She needs to move around; if she lies too long, she could get a block in her leg veins.'

Next time, Nellie had arisen, but the apron-clad Edward

11

was obviously going to remain cook and parlourmaid to her ladyship, whatever I said.

He came to the door with me and stood looking out at the view. The wind from the west riffled through the shining, uncut grass of the fields. 'Luvly, in't it, doctor? Nellie and me did a lot of our courtin' in them medders, just after the war. I was 'ere convalescin', stayed on too an' got a job, store-keepin', never went back to London no more.'

'Yes, it's lovely, Edward.'

He sniffed the wind. 'Didn't get air like this in the Old Kent Road. Never mind it rattlin' the winders. Nellie ain't so keen though, likes it nice and balmy-like.'

As I got into my car I noticed a thin, elderly man in a black Homburg hat and tired, pin-stripe black suit coming slowly along the footpath. He looked away when he saw me.

I wondered idly who he was. He looked like an undertaker, but he wasn't one I knew from the town.

It was several weeks before I saw the Gascoignes again. Nellie didn't come to the surgery as she had promised, and I was too busy to chase up patients who didn't do what they were asked. We were in the middle of the hectic holiday period at Wilverton. Added to the work of summer visitors who ate too many winkles, stayed too long in the sun or got stung by jelly-fish, we were always one man short in the practice: one of us – Charles Semple, Fred Wilson or myself – would take time off in turn.

The Hamilton bank account was oscillating in and out of the red danger zone, so, with the boarding-school bills of the two boys coming up, there didn't look like being any going away this year. Peter and Barney couldn't have cared less – being home was holiday enough for them. After all, we were already by the south coast and what they wanted to do most was to muck about in our assorted craft, which ranged from a float (bought second-hand from the Corporation Amusements) to an elderly canoe and the dinghy Charles had once built for me. All Sarah asked was to tag along.

By united efforts we had practically rebuilt a derelict hut on a distant, quiet beach. We shared the beach-hut with Charles, but as he was away, we could now have it all to

12

ourselves. As often as possible I would take all the family down there for a picnic lunch, snatch a bathe myself and keep in touch with the surgery through a handy telephone kiosk. I would do my visits and call back for them in time to get to evening surgery.

Miss Spencer, our faithful secretary, answered the phone this time. 'Yes, doctor, there are two visits. One is for Mrs Gascoigne – I should go there first. The other's a bit odd. It's Mrs Bamford – you know, doctor, the Baptist minister's wife. She wants to talk to you urgently and she can't come to the surgery for some reason.'

'That's OK. We'll cope. Ring me at the Bamfords' if you need me. 'Bye.'

As I reached the gate of the Gascoignes' terrace-house, there was the thin man in the Homburg again. This time he was hurrying out, and he brushed past me almost rudely. Edward seemed ill at ease. He forgot to shake hands.

'Nellie's bad again, doctor. I'm that sorry she didn't coom ter see you.'

She was right back where we started – only worse. This time there were definite signs of heart failure. The rosy cheeks had a bluish tinge and her breathlessness was real. Her ankles weren't only fat, they dented when I pressed them. I didn't try any drastic remedies but put her back on her tablets straight away and added something to relieve the fluid retention.

She looked away when I asked her questions and did not answer. I was mystified. There seemed to be a barrier between us. In the hall I had to tell Edward that his wife was much more ill than she had been before. He squeezed my arm. 'Do yer best for her, doctor, she's all I got.'

I had to pass the village shop on my way back, so I popped in to get a block of ice cream for the family. After all, as they weren't getting a proper holiday they could do with a little treat.

It was a pleasant, old-fashioned general store. I moved through the sacks of vegetables, the stacks of tinned food and floor-brushes to the corner where there were cooked meats and a refrigerator with the ice creams. I paid the lady

13

behind the counter and was turning to leave when she stopped me.

'Doctor, could I have a word? I'm Mr Gascoigne's niece.' I had that other visit to the Bamfords' to do but I paused. There was something troubling her, that was obvious.

'. . . Perhaps I shouldn't interfere, but Aunt Nellie . . . did you know she's been seeing another doctor?' So that was it. She plunged on. 'I call him a "doctor", but he's just a quack. That's why she hasn't been to see you.'

'What's his name?' I asked.

'Frinton, Dr Frinton.'

'Who's he? I don't know any doctor round here called that.'

'He's a horrible little man in a black suit.'

The thin man in the Homburg! Frinton? . . . Frinton . . . Now I remembered. Fred had told me, but it was years before . . . I had always pictured a man rather like the East Coast resort of the same name – genteel, associated with the acting profession, and not in the least like the shifty-looking customer I had twice encountered. Fred, generous to a fault, had told me, more in sorrow than indignation, that the said 'Frinton' had been struck off for serious malpractice, a patient had nearly died. . .

Miss Gascoigne was still talking: 'He's got a real hold on Auntie, reckons he's curing her with his hypnotism and herbs, and Uncle has to give in to her. That's why she hasn't come back to you before.'

'Don't do anything about it, Miss Gascoigne. I'll fix it tomorrow, I promise you. I've got to go and see another patient now, but thank you for telling me. You did the right thing.'

Mrs Bamford led me into the shabby little lounge of the Baptist manse and sat down with her head bowed. Her hands were trembling; she pressed the palms together between her knees. The story came out bit by bit: their shortage of money, the demands the church work made on her husband, James, the snide remarks she would overhear if he ever suggested that something was too much for him to undertake.

14

He was out every night in the week at meetings; he was always so busy that he hardly had time to eat his meals and just flopped into bed at night with hardly a 'Good-night'. She would wake to find him in the kitchen making tea because he couldn't sleep with so much on his mind, and he would snap at her or the children over trifles, in a most uncharacteristic way. He would come and apologize afterwards, but she knew he couldn't help it.

But what was really worrying her was that on more than one occasion recently he had been half-way through a sermon and then had suddenly stopped, become red and confused and brought his theme to an obviously inconclusive halt. Once, afterwards, he had told her that his mind had simply gone blank.

'I'm so worried about him, doctor. Could you give him a pick-me-up or should he consult a psychiatrist? I feel I should be praying more for him.' Her chin trembled as she finished speaking.

'Mrs Bamford, it's not more prayer he needs – it's a holiday. If he doesn't get away, he'll have a breakdown. Please tell him – whatever he's got booked for tonight, he must get someone to stand in for him. I'll come back and have a chat with him; it really is urgent. Will you tell him that from me?'

As I drove away, I was thinking what a dangerous authority we doctors assume over our patients and what a lonely life a minister has, always expected to be on top spiritual form, with maybe only his doctor to share his self-doubt and feelings of inadequacy with. However, my more immediate worry was that it was very nearly surgery time and Elisabeth and the children would be waiting anxiously for me to pick them up. When we got home, I had just time for a quick cup and then I was off to surgery.

When I looked in at the manse afterwards, I put my proposition of a holiday to James Bamford. He had sacrificed a deacons' meeting to wait for me. 'But if I suddenly pack it in, it will look like a victory for the devil!' he protested.

'But it will be a far greater victory for him if you collapse

15

in church – and that's what you're heading for, if you don't let up.'

He grinned, and he began to lose the harried look just a little. 'We-ell, I have got a sister married to a farmer down in Somerset. We'd be welcome to stay there for a week and we'd love it.'

'*Three* weeks or even four – no less,' I said firmly.

'You win, doctor, we'll do it. After all, if I haven't been able to train some of my flock to act as temporary shepherds by now, I'd better pack it in anyway!'

When I got home I asked Elisabeth how the kids had enjoyed the ice cream.

'It wasn't bad through a straw,' she said.

Before I got through into the temporary ground-floor bedroom next day, Edward Gascoigne had confessed that Nellie had always been such a one for the miracle-workers, that when a neighbour had sung the praises of 'Doctor' Frinton, she'd insisted that Edward call him in.

'Three quid! Three bloomin' quid, that's what he charged us for every visit. Knocked a sockin' great 'ole in my post office account, 'e 'as. That's why she never kime ter see yer and why she wouldn't let me send. I'm that sorry, doctor; 'im an' 'is blinkin' 'erbs 'an 'is "Watch the pendulum, my dear"! Fat lot of good they've done.'

I got the gentleman's telephone number from Edward (I'd already discovered that he was ex-directory) and that night I rang him and told him in no uncertain terms what would happen to him if he interfered with Nellie or any other of my patients again.

Despite her serious relapse, Nellie seemed to be picking up nicely. Then suddenly, around six o'clock one evening, an emergency call came through. I had to leave a surgery half-full of patients which Charles, now back from his holiday, manfully took over, but by the time I got to the terrace-house overlooking the fields, she had gone. One of those hardened arteries had blocked and her sorely strained heart had given up. The sun had gone down and the evening wind was rattling the windows as I pulled the sheet back over her quiet face.

Edward was walking about as in a dream. He had on his apron as usual and his poor right hand clutched and twisted at it. I put an arm round his shoulders and we knelt as I prayed for his comfort and commended Nellie to a heavenly Father's care. His niece came in and I left to ring up the undertaker on his behalf.

Some lines of poetry I only half knew were tweaking my memory as I drove home – some lines about 'the west wind'. Before I could sit down to the meal Elisabeth had ready for me, I searched an old anthology and found they were Shelley's. Strangely appropriate they were too, and in his 'Ode to the West Wind':

> As thus with thee in prayer in my sore need,
> Oh lift me as a wave, a leaf, a cloud!
> I fall upon the thorns of life! I bleed!

The gold had gone completely from the sky – and I thought sadly that the gold had gone out of Edward's life too. No celebration of fifty years of marriage for him now. The gallant little man with a maimed hand who had survived a bitter war and lived to look after his beloved Nellie for nearly fifty years no longer had anything to keep him. A month later I was finding it difficult to find a cause to put on *his* death certificate. The registrar will not accept 'Sorrow and Age' as adequate.

One Sunday, I forsook Wilverton Parish Church and went to the Baptist Church for the evening service. A relaxed and bronzed minister delivered a powerful address with no awkward pauses. His handshake at the door was positively painful.

2
It never rains . . .

Monday morning . . . half past six . . . I got up and pulled the curtains back. There was nothing to suggest that the immediate future held any particular menace. No feeling of impending crisis weighed me down. True, the skies outside were dark and glowering – but they had been like that all the past week. What else should one expect at the height of an English summer?

Elisabeth's voice broke the silence, her tones muffled by the bedclothes. 'Going to make the tea, love?'

I bent over her and kissed her forehead, the only part of her face visible. 'That was my intention. What sort would you like?' (We allow ourselves one definite luxury: we do like decent tea – not strong, but good quality and varied, with just a few grains of sugar, a fair dash of milk, a heated pot *and* china cups – good big ones. Ours don't match; coming from Wilverton market stalls it would be unlikely that they would, but that doesn't spoil the pleasure of drinking from them.)

As I waited for the kettle to boil I felt no sense of oppression though I did have a slight headache. Our time of Bible reading and prayer was undramatic. No words of warning stood out from the Bible page; we felt no dynamic urgency as we prayed together over the day. Our customary routine moved ahead in well-oiled fashion. At breakfast Elisabeth plied me with my usual orange juice, porridge, slice of lean bacon and one piece of toast and marmalade. Sarah cycled off to school, joined by her friend from down the road. I left for the surgery in a serene frame of mind.

It was all too normal. There at the head of the queue was the familiar figure of Mrs Bennett waiting for her regular injection for pernicious anaemia. Mrs Bennett has a peculiar gift for conducting her own private drama session, taking both parts in the dialogue. Today she ran strictly to form.

'I said to Ben, "This is my injection day, this is."

' "Are you sure dear?"

' "Yes, it's always the day I change the library books."

' "I thought that was last week."

' "Don't be a goose, that was the day for the dog food."

' "All right then, you can get me some tobacco from the newsagents' when you're passing."

' "I wish you'd stop that horrid habit, Ben, I can't stand it."

' "Well, you've put up with it for forty years, why are you complaining now?"

' "I'm going to ask the doctor. I'm sure it's doing your lungs no good."

' "Now don't you go bothering doctor about things like that. He's got enough to do as it is."

' "I shall, you see if I don't." '

I finished the injection, shook her by the hand and said, 'Tell Mr Bennett that smoking doesn't do him any good – but don't go and make trouble, will you?'

Her voice, a level monotone, faded down the passage. 'I shall say "Ben, what did I tell you? Doctor says smoking does you harm. . ." '

The first signs of the gathering storm would have been picked up by a more discerning eye than mine at the entry in the visiting book at the end of the morning's surgery session. Strange, I thought, to have a call from the Boys' Home when I had been there for my weekly checks only the day before.

I found Tommy pale and shocked, lying on his bed in the dormitory.

'Called me in the night,' said the superintendent, 'Uncle John' to the boys. 'Said he'd a pain in his side. Didn't seem too bad so I gave him an aspirin, but he was worse this morning.'

Tommy certainly had something unusual. As I passed my hand over his side he cringed and pushed my hand away. His right knee was a little swollen and he wouldn't move it.

19

''Urts, doctor,' he whispered. He had a moderate rise in temperature.

I pulled the bedclothes right down. The pieces of jigsaw began to fit together – he had red spots over his shins . . . Purpura! Henoch's Purpura. I beckoned to Uncle John who followed me out on to the landing.

'That lad should be in hospital. He's got a kind of allergic reaction which causes blood to pass through the small blood vessels into the kidney, knee joints and skin. That's what's causing his pain and these blotches. It could be dangerous and he must be under observation.'

'Allergic to what, doctor? He hasn't had anything unusual.'

'It could be a bug. Has he had a sore throat at all?'

'He did have a bit of one two days ago, but it didn't seem anything to worry about.'

The ambulance men picked up the anxious-looking scrap of humanity. As they were lifting him carefully on to the stretcher I said, 'Soon be back home, Tommy, we'll play football together again.' He smiled a wan little smile.

All this made a big hole in my day and I'd got an anaesthetic to give for a dentist in the centre of town at half past twelve. I made it with a few minutes to spare. As I entered the waiting-room there was 'Corp', (short for 'Corporal', as the boys called him), Uncle John's right-hand man at the Boys' Home.

'Can't get away from you lot,' I said. 'What's your trouble?' I needn't really have asked – his left cheek was badly swollen. He pointed at it ruefully. The gas went well, though Corp took longer than usual to come round.

'How are you getting home?' I asked, as we went outside.

'Bus,' he mumbled, through a handkerchief.

'I'll give you a lift – it's on my way,' I said.

Corp sat in the front holding his blood-stained hanky to his mouth. Half-way home I glanced across at him. He was leaning forward with beads of sweat standing out on his forehead.

'You all right, Corp?'

He could only shake his head, then, 'Feel sick,' he gasped.

I pulled the car to the side of the road, leapt out and opened the boot. Thank goodness, I'd got the new dustbin I'd bought for Elisabeth still in there unshipped. I grabbed the lid, tore open the passenger door and thrust it on to Corp's knees. He bowed his head over it in abject misery. We stopped again by a little copse just down the road from the Boys' Home and I emptied the lid into the undergrowth. Corp was regaining his normal colour by the time we reached the house. He got out of the car and staggered inside. Somehow lunch wasn't so appetizing that day.

I had no more visits, so I booked an appointment at the barber's and went to get a haircut. (My colleague Charles Semple, had been making one or two snide remarks about 'long-haired lay-abouts' so I'd taken the hint.) I thought I could relax for a spell in the chair without fear of the telephone. Mr Semproni, alias 'Bert Smith' – another patient of ours – always had a soothing effect on me. As he clipped away, there was no need for me to do more than emit an occasional 'Mm', 'Really?', 'Uh-huh', while his stream of conversation proceeded unhindered. It was chiefly about hairdressing, how it combined an art and a craft and should be classed as a profession, not a trade.

Suddenly I was aware of a lull. The scissors no longer snipped, the soporific flow of verbiage had ceased abruptly. I opened my eyes. In the mirror I couldn't even *see* Mr Semproni. He had disappeared. I wheeled round in the chair, nearly strangling myself as the sheet round my neck caught on its arms, and there he was, curled up on the floor, his face contorted and his fingers clutching his midriff, his scissors and comb lying beside him.

'What on earth's the matter?' I cried.

'Pain – in me side.' He barely got it out through his clenched teeth. His knees were almost up to his chest and he was writhing to and fro. I jumped across to the shop door, slammed it shut and pulled down the blind. Kneeling down by Mr Semproni, I gently examined him. The only likely explanation of his sudden collapse in pain was a stone in his right ureter, the tube that runs from the kidney to the bladder.

21

'Hold on a moment, just hold on.' It was rather a silly thing to say – there wasn't much else he could do.

I wrenched open the door and ran round to my car which was parked in a side road. In a minute I was back with my bag, though on the way I got some peculiar looks from passers-by. They couldn't have been used to seeing a man in a hair-cutting sheet running wildly along the pavement.

I gave him a big shot of pethidine and used his telephone to call an ambulance. Dropping the latch to his shop on my way out, I left for home as unobtrusively as possible. I wasn't too keen to be seen again in public. I had removed the sheet but I was moderately well known in the town and my hair-cut – completed on one side only – might have given the impression that the local GP had joined some strange new cult. Elisabeth gave me remedial care between bursts of uncontrollable mirth.

It was odd to have had two abdominal crises in the one day – Tommy and now my barber, although Tommy really had a much more generalized condition. Evening surgery was the heaviest it had been for some time. I was beginning to realize that this was going to be a week to remember – or perhaps a week I'd rather forget.

I saw Tommy in hospital the next day and was sad to learn that his condition was worse. He did not smile at me this time. His notes revealed that he was now passing blood in his motions.

Corp's wife, Sylvia, was due for a final antenatal examination on the Wednesday of that week, but she didn't turn up. Instead, there was a message from the midwife to say that she had gone into labour a week early. Although it was her first, she and Corp had insisted that the birth should take place at home. 'Home' was a little cottage attached to the main building of the Boys' Home. The midwife had said she would call me when I was needed. I was – at 11.35 p.m. The baby's head was just showing. A quarter of an hour later, Corp had a new recruit.

We waited and waited but the placenta refused to come. Sylvia was losing a lot of blood and I was worried. In Africa, with no other help at hand, I would have gone ahead and removed the afterbirth manually, but here, with sterile conditions, good anaesthesia and blood transfusions available close by in hospital, I felt the risk was unjustified. We called the ambulance yet again and she was taken in to the maternity unit at the local hospital.

'Getting a bit of a habit, isn't it, doc?' said the ambulance man over his shoulder as he climbed in. I learned later that she needed two pints of blood before the job was complete.

Thursday and Friday were busy days, but there were no alarms or excursions. Tommy's condition was still pretty serious.

Saturday drifted by – surgery, visits and a phone-call to the hospital, who told me, to my great relief, that Tommy was out of danger. I sat down to a high tea in a happier frame of mind and with a more voracious appetite than I'd had all week. Elisabeth had just handed me a nicely grilled local plaice when the phone rang. It was 'Uncle John's voice.

'Sorry, doctor, but I've got more trouble.'

'Not another boy like Tommy, surely?'

'You won't believe it, it's Corp. He's in a right state.'

I did find it hard to believe. He was usually as hard as nails, and apart from our one little episode with the dustbin lid after the tooth extraction, he had never required medical assistance. Football with the boys, working in the grounds, general maintenance, on top of all his routine work as a housemaster – he was always hard at it, cheerful and tireless. I had been surprised, I now recalled, at his upset over a little thing like an anaesthetic.

'He wouldn't be having a stomach-ache by any chance, would he?' I said sarcastically, remembering our home-help Mrs Clout's aphorism: 'Troubles always come in threes.' (Or fours, I thought, counting Sylvia.)

'Clever of you, doc. He's doubled up. Got him in bed, and he's been sick too – all over the place. Started feeling poorly this morning but he thought it would pass off. I'd be grateful if you'd look in.'

When I examined him there wasn't a shadow of doubt: Corp had an acute appendicitis, and he'd be lucky if he hadn't perforated into the bargain. The ambulance super-

23

visor sounded incredulous when I made my call. 'Have to charge you by the dozen, doctor.'

It had been *quite* a week, but that was the last spot of bother, and on Sunday, my free day, Elisabeth, Sarah and I went to church and I said a special 'thank you' that my casualties were all doing well. Corp hadn't perforated after all.

24

3

Sauce for the gander

I suppose if anyone is to blame it must be my father. My memory of him is of a lovable but austere and impatient Scot who did what he thought was right, irrespective of anyone else's opinions. My mother told me that from the start of their life together he would carry nonconformity to extremes. He felt that Scottish law was superior to English – and this conviction caused my mother a lot of unnecessary trouble later on. He died young and the will had to be administered in Scotland; by then we had moved to England, so this was a difficult and costly business.

When I came to join the family circle, he wouldn't have me christened or vaccinated. I didn't know the difference at the time, but later he wouldn't agree for me to have my tonsils out. Having remedied the first two omissions, I was now suffering from the last.

'I really must give Saunders a ring about my throat,' I said hoarsely to Elisabeth.

'Yes, dear,' she said, and went on sewing.

I was a bit hurt. I felt she might have shown some concern – here was I, always fit, having to see a medical man and a surgeon at that.

'It'll mean going in for an op.' I added plaintively.

'Yes, dear, better get it over with,' was all I got in response to my attempts to tug at the heart-strings.

'You aren't showing much sympathy, are you?' I couldn't help saying.

Elisabeth looked up at me with a smile that said, 'You are a big baby', but her words were, 'It'll only be for a few days, won't it? You've been moaning about it for ages, it's about time something was done.' Coming from someone who'd had three children and three major operations that was pretty reasonable, so I shut up and went off to phone Saunders.

Our ear, nose and throat consultant is a no-nonsense type.

'Of course I'll have to see you first, Hamilton. If they need to come out, 'fraid I haven't a bed at the moment at the D.O.G.S.', (the insalubrious abbreviation for the Duke of Gloucester's Sanatorium, our local district hospital), 'but I could probably fit you in at the Brendon Cottage Hospital.'

'That'll be fine,' I said.

'Right then. Come and see me on Tuesday at 2.30; you'll only be in for a few days.'

So there I was, complete with bag containing pyjamas, toothbrush, shaving kit and a large book, waiting at the door of the ward, feeling rather like a lion about to enter a den of Daniels.

Sister Marjorie was giving out duties to her nursing staff. At last she turned and saw me.

'Oh, doctor, sorry to keep you waiting. I've put you in a side-room but you'll have to share it. We're full up on the ward and we had a burns case come in yesterday, so we've had to put him in with you.'

I've seen some odd-looking specimens in my time, but my room-mate took the biscuit – and a burnt biscuit at that. His face, which seemed naturally a deep brown, was patched all over with areas of blackened skin, and his hair and beard were singed off to a straggly stubble.

'Mr Gadsby,' said Nurse Esther, 'this is Doctor Hamilton who is going to share your room.' His eyes flicked up to mine for a second and then looked away. He nodded.

'Sorry to butt in on you,' I said. 'I hope you're feeling better today after your accident?' I automatically assumed my slightly superior medical tones. But Mr Gadsby didn't seem to notice. He just nodded again.

Between the sister's office and the door of the side-ward, the nurse had told me quickly that Gadsby was a tramp who had accidentally set himself on fire while brewing tea in a barn. He had been lucky not to burn down the whole barn but had, in fact, apparently bravely put himself and the

26

lighted straw out before calling for help. The staff obviously had a soft spot for him.

Although in the side-ward, he was like a frightened rabbit and seldom said anything. I could see that our sojourn together was unlikely to be a riotous one but perhaps that was just as well – it would give my throat a rest and enable me to get down to the biography of Lister, the great innovator in antiseptic surgery. If hardly light relief, I reckoned it would occupy my mind.

And yet, I found that Gadsby – odd as he was – immediately fascinated me. He was a loner; maybe he *had* opted out, but perhaps he saw things the rest of us were missing in our rush through life. If I could win his confidence, he might open up – though if I had a couple of ragged holes in my throat by tomorrow where my tonsils had been, I mightn't be feeling too much like conversation. Still, I could try *listening*, something I'm always meaning to do. (Hadn't the apostle Paul said something about 'buying up opportunities'?) Perhaps we'd been thrown together for some reason. . .

The needle slid slickly into my bulging forearm vein. Through his mask the anaesthetist told me to count up to ten. (He sounded slightly bored, but he might just have been partly anaesthetized himself from anaesthetics breathed on him by earlier patients.) I obeyed. 'One, two, thre-ee, fo. . . Surely there shouldn't be a spider stalking along the cornice of a hospital ward? I shifted my head to get a better look. Ouch! A small dagger stabbed me in the tonsils. Tonsils? I swallowed; it felt like broken glass. It sank in – they're out, it's all over!

I focussed carefully on the figure in the chair across the room. Then I remembered: Gadsby! He actually spoke – and he had quite a cultured voice.

'How do you feel? I was wondering when you would come round.'

I didn't try answering. I just stuck my thumb in the air. He grinned. Nurse Esther came in with a jug and poured out a drink for me. I sipped it gratefully – it was iced water. Swallowing it wasn't too bad.

I croaked out, 'Nurse, I'm starving.'

She smiled. 'Only slops for you today. Do you fancy some jelly and ice cream?'

To my chagrin, when it arrived about an hour later, I didn't really fancy food after all. In fact, I was beginning to feel 'proper poorly' – all shivery and headachy. When the coast was clear, I reached out and picked the thermometer out of its little jar of pink fluid from my bedside cabinet and stuck it in my mouth.

'Here, you shouldn't be doing that,' said Gadsby reprovingly. 'They won't let me take mine.' I grinned feebly and held up a finger to my lips.

When I thought it was cooked, I read the thermometer. 103.4! No wonder I wasn't feeling so good. I put the thermometer back, pulled the bedclothes up to my chin and had a think.

It would have been better if I hadn't taken my temperature. All the most gruesome possibilities now began coursing through my fevered brain. Then my teeth began to chatter and I knew I was having a genuine rigor. When the nurse came to take our temperatures, she took one look at mine, recorded it on the chart and departed swiftly.

The house surgeon came in about a couple of minutes later and examined me. He said nothing, but he too went away at once, looking worried. It wasn't long before he was back. He made a good effort to look unconcerned.

'You've got a bit of a fever,' he said nonchalantly. 'I've had a word with Mr Saunders on the phone; he advises some aspirin and a sedative.' I felt slightly demeaned but secretly, I was comforted. Couldn't be too bad if Saunders wasn't bothered.

After the aspirin I felt somewhat less lousy but during the night I sweated, turned and ached all over. I vowed I wouldn't be so sceptical in future with patients who say, 'Doctor, I didn't sleep a wink last night!' The nurses blanket-bathed me three times, and changed me from my own pyjamas to hospital flannelette ones with great patience.

When daylight came at last, I was lying exhausted. Gadsby stirred at last and opened his eyes. He stared at me for a moment. 'Doctor, you don't half look funny!'

I managed, 'You don't look so wonderful yourself', before my throat gave out.

'No, I mean you really do. You're all spotty, like measles.'

'I've had measles,' I grated.

Someone had left a hand-mirror by the wash-basin. Gadsby shuffled across, picked it up and handed it to me with his bandaged fingers. I got a glimpse of my face and neck and then my medical awareness took over.

'You'd better keep right away from me,' I said, thinking of his burns area. 'I think I've got scarlet fever.'

'Not to worry,' he said quite cheerfully, 'I've had that.'

'Better give the bell a ring,' I whispered hoarsely.

That did it. It was like letting off a firework in a hen-run. The entire hospital staff seemed to commence running to and fro. The nurses who now approached us were gowned and masked like Arab houris. Sister stood before me, her eyes hot and indignant above her veil. 'A proper disaster area you are, doctor! We'll have to close the hospital.' I felt this fell short of the standard of dispassionate care one expects of a dedicated profession, but in the circumstances I felt it wiser not to mention it.

Saunders came at two o'clock, none too pleased, I guess, at having to cut short his lunch-break. He looked at me.

'Strep. infection. Must have come in with it. Give him penicillin injections – should clear up quickly.'

I gurgled apologetically, 'I'm sorry, Mr Saunders. I'm sensitive to penicillin. It brings me out in spots.' That sounded particularly ridiculous in the circumstances.

Saunders' look said plainly, 'We've got a right one here', but his actual words were, 'Well, give him Erythromycin,' and I guess he also ordered a shot of morphia, when he heard of my previous night. Despite the morphia, I didn't sleep again, but I was free from the worst of the pain and I didn't care.

As the night ticked slowly by, I tried praying but my mind wandered all over the place. In the darkened room I looked across at Gadsby snoring peacefully and thought, 'I'm glad you're enjoying a short spell of human care and comfort in your self-chosen existence.' Then I thought about Jesus who, in his time on earth, 'had nowhere to lay his head'.

I felt well enough next day to pick up my New Testament. It was a copy of the translation by J. B. Phillips. I caught Gadsby looking at me. He had woken up but hadn't made a move. After a moment he said quietly, 'Get anything out of that?'

'Yes,' I answered. 'Directions for the day.'

He grunted and then lay still for some minutes. Then, without warning, he began to talk freely. 'You won't believe this, doctor, but when I was a boy I once thought seriously about becoming a parson.' He looked shyly at me to see the effect of this announcement. I said nothing.

After a pause he went on: 'I left school, went on to tech to get some more exams, you know. Had a nice girl-friend too . . .' He spoke in staccato sentences, leaving me to fill in the gaps. 'Then . . . Mum and Dad died . . . killed, both of them, in the Midlands train smash. Just after that, my girl deserted me for a school pal of mine – well, I *thought* he was a pal,' he added bitterly. 'Couldn't see where God fitted into a situation like that, so I left the tech. Left home too, and went on the road. Been on the move ever since – ten years I suppose, 'til this lot . . . why am I telling you all this?'

There was a silence. 'Ever think about God again?' I asked.

He shook his head, then, 'Well, once, it was up north. I remember, I kipped for the night in the crypt of a church – St George's, in Leeds. They were really good to me – made me think a bit. I guess you believe in God, don't you?'

'Yes, I do,' I said.

There was another silence. I wondered if his spate of confidentiality had spent itself. I thought he was flushing under that mottling of burnt skin. All morning I thought over what he'd confided to me. Gadsby was no ordinary tramp – but what is an 'ordinary tramp' anyway? I wondered whether I'd better let the whole business drop, if it embarrassed him so much. But, on the other hand, if he'd been a patient in the surgery, I wouldn't just have passed the whole thing up. Wasn't his telling me a *cri de coeur* that I shouldn't ignore? Something had made him share his secret with me.

There must be some bond that he felt between us but I must respect his feelings and tread with the greatest care.

After lunch I broke the silence. 'Gadsby, what's your Christian name? It seems silly calling each other 'Gadsby' and 'Doctor' when we're shoved together like this.'

'Arnold,' he said, a little grudgingly.

After a few minutes I tried again. 'Arnold, it's difficult for me to imagine how you felt, losing everyone you loved at once like that. That's never happened to me.' He just nodded. 'It must have seemed like the end of the world . . . no wonder you wanted to break everything up, go away and forget it all.' I waited but he made no response. 'You haven't forgotten though, have you?' He shook his head. 'I don't suppose you've come up with any answers either. Have you ever felt that perhaps you pushed God out too quickly, didn't really give him a chance?'

There was another long pause, but he was looking at me with a sort of hopeless hunger in his eyes. It was all uphill but I had to keep going. 'D'you think it might just be that he allowed these tragedies because he had to know if you would keep trusting him, whatever happened, just like Job in the Bible? I haven't suffered like you, Arnold, but I did have to chuck up my whole career in Africa because of illness and I've found God all the more important to me through it.' I stopped, wondering if I'd already said too much.

It turned out to be a busy day. After lunch, which I really enjoyed, Charles brought Elisabeth to see me. He stood at the end of my bed, looking through the bottom half of his bifocals at my four-hourly temperature chart. It had mercifully settled from a series of mountain peaks to a comfortable plateau.

'Hmmm. Trust you to make the most of a simple thing like a tonsillectomy,' he said, in his usual comforting manner. Then, from behind his back he produced a big bunch of beautiful sweet peas. 'Lilian sent you these to sweeten you up a bit.' I knew they were his own prize blooms. Contacts with Charles are always bracing. I began to feel distinctly better. 'I'll leave you to Elisabeth's tender care now.' He turned towards the door. 'I'll be outside in the car. Don't

31

be too long, I've got some visits to finish.' Elisabeth nodded obediently.

When he'd gone she produced two bunches of beautiful black grapes from a bag. She went over to Arnold and held out one.

'Would you like these, Mr Gadsby?' she said smiling. I'd told her a bit about my room-mate the night I came in, on the telephone. He didn't reply but simply nodded his head. The look in his eyes as he took them made me think of a dog getting a pat from a stranger he wasn't quite sure of.

She placed the remaining bunch in the dish by my bed, sat down and began telling me quietly how much she and the children were missing me, especially as it was holiday-time, all about the garden and one or two patients who had rung up enquiring about me and when I would be back.

'We miss you a lot, darling,' she whispered at the end. Then, out loud, 'Have to go, mustn't keep Charles waiting. Goodbye love, goodbye Mr Gadsby, don't let my husband bully you.' For a moment his face lit up and he grinned.

Over the next few days my temperature stayed flat and normal and I began to feel really well. Conversation with Arnold was rather one-way traffic – either he didn't answer or did so in monosyllables. One morning, the houseman told me that Mr Saunders had said that if I was still OK I could go home the next day.

In the morning I was stuffing my possessions into my bag when I had a thought. I went over to Arnold and held out my New Testament. 'I'd like you to have this as a memento of our spell of confinement together; please take it.' I shook his bandaged hand with care. 'Thank you,' was all he said.

To my chagrin I found that the practice was progressing very nicely in my absence and, as if to emphasize this, Charles rang up the day after my return home to assure me, 'No need to hurry back, old chap, take all the time you want. We don't want you flopping out again as soon as you get back to work. The locum we've got' (he was newly qualified from Barts'), 'is doing very well. In fact, he gets through about twice your usual amount.'

This was in Charles's normal reassuring vein, but I read

between the lines. No locum, however efficient, can avoid being a bit of a headache. He doesn't know the patients or their families, he doesn't know the district and he either thinks he knows too much or is very unsure of himself. So I knew that this was really Charles's backhanded but kind way of saying I was to take my time.

However, as I was paying the locum fees and my sickness insurance didn't really cover them, I was keen to return as soon as possible. I was surprisingly weak on my pins still, so I was glad to take another week off. Elisabeth's cooking was working wonders. The hospital food hadn't been too bad, but I did wish that it hadn't all been steamed in washing-up cloths before serving.

We thought about Gadsby often in the next week or so, especially after we had enquired about him soon after I returned home and found he had discharged himself before he was due to go and the hospital hadn't a clue as to his whereabouts.

I was reading the daily paper after lunch about eighteen months later when my eye caught a short paragraph at the bottom of the middle page. It was headed, 'Gallantry of a Gentleman of the Road, from our West of England correspondent.'

'From a statement issued by the police at Crewkerne, we learn of the death in tragic circumstances of an unknown vagrant. When questioned, Mr E. G. Bailey, who farms 200 acres a mile or so from the town, confirmed that he had employed a tramp as casual labour. "He seemed a decent enough bloke and we needed an extra hand temporarily." This man came to the rescue of Mr Bailey when he had been felled by his Friesian bull in the yard. Sadly, he too was knocked down by the bull while fending it off Mr Bailey, and was fatally gored. There were no papers on this brave wayfarer to enable the police to identify him and inform any next of kin. The only thing found on him was a well-worn New Testament in modern English. "He gave the name of Gadsby," stated Mr Bailey. "But I didn't think that was likely to be his real name." Attempts to discover who he was are continuing.'

4

'A being darkly wise'

Almost without our noticing it the years had drifted by and Africa now lay far behind us. It wasn't that we never thought of those years in a small mission hospital, high in the mountains of Kenya. If it hadn't been for ill-health in the family, we would have been there still, and we had never lost our love for the land or its peoples.

But, if we'd imagined that being buried in the hinterland of the British establishment would shut out Africa, we would have been mistaken – and very happily mistaken at that. We'd left Africa, but Africa refused to leave us. For one thing, our local College of Further Education attracted students from all over the world, including Africa. Nigerians from the west, Arabs from the north, Asians and tribal folk from the east – they all came to Wilverton, and many came to our surgery as well, as they fell victim to the products of the British scene: colds and 'flu and tonsillitis *and* loneliness.

Now and then there were other contacts which brought on bouts of acute nostalgia in us.

The phone rang one day, and a Kenyan friend was at the other end of the line.

'Would you like to have Benjamin, son of Abraham, to tea?'

For a moment I thought he'd got his millenia and his genealogy in a twist! Then I remembered a little boy in patched khaki shorts and little else, holding the hand of his father, Abraham, one of our schoolteachers, a man who had only reached a standard or two above his son.

'Rather,' I said, 'but what is he doing in England?'

'Oh, just a bit of post-graduate research in anthropology at Cambridge,' he replied.

Benjamin was delightful. Our daughter, Sarah, put him at

his ease and they were soon deep in conversation, as she really loved geography. Very courteously he corrected her grammar once or twice, and I heard him encouraging her to persevere in her studies. We sat him at the tea-table in the window where he could look out towards the Downs beyond the trees at the bottom of our garden. It was the nearest we could offer to the vastnesses at the door of his old home that we too had known so well. Later we received a copy of the book he had written on the history and customs of his branch of the Kalenjin ethnic group.

Then one day a few months later, a young Ugandan Asian came to the surgery. I thought he was a student, but he was actually a business man who had come for a life insurance examination. Youthful he might be, but he was buying premises in Wilverton to set up a shop. It seemed he was continuing a family tradition. 'My father keeps a shop back at home in Fort Portal,' he told me.

A nephew of ours was in charge of a hospital nearby. Out of interest we wrote to him and asked if he knew the young man's father. 'Know him?' came the reply. 'He owns half the town!'

We realized that the son had come on ahead while the going was good to set up a new base of operations. Sure enough, Amin's reign of terror would come before long to Uganda, with disastrous consequences for the country's Asian population.

Africa would simply not leave us alone! I couldn't get to a medical society meeting one evening, so, sure enough, I was proposed, seconded and carried (kicking) into the membership of a committee of the NHS GP Appointments, there being no other candidates for this prestigious but unpaid post.

Soon we had to choose someone to fill a practice vacancy in another part of Wilverton. Three doctors were short-listed. One's qualifications, though impressive, were found, by calculating the dates of their attainment, to be fictitious, so he was eliminated. Of the remaining two, the first had experience and degrees far superior to the second; he was a Dr Awolo from Nigeria. I at once proposed his acceptance

35

but I had not reckoned with the opposition. Natterby, a member of Wilverton Town Council, interposed. His qualifications for the committee were ownership of an amusement arcade, plus a series of betting shops along the south coast.

'I've no prejudice myself against coloured people, but what are our missuses going to say? How will they like having a blackie examine them?' I didn't wholly blame him for his fears of the unfamiliar, but before I could reply through the chairman, the matter was taken out of my hands.

A bus inspector who was a union shop-steward, another member of the committee, jumped in. 'Well, *my* missus wouldn't mind for a start. What matters is – is he a good doctor? Bloomin' racial prejudice, that's what it is!' (Only he didn't say 'bloomin''.)

Dr Awolo was appointed and soon became one of the most popular and efficient doctors in the town.

It wasn't so much that Elisabeth and I were Anglophobes – we were Afrophiles. But not every touch with those hailing from the misnamed 'Dark Continent' left me unscathed. . .

The atmosphere in the operating theatre at the D.O.G.S. seemed more oppressive than in the theatres I remembered from my own hospital days. Surreptitiously I wiped my face on the sleeve of my gown; I was only observing, not assisting, after all. I sucked my breath in through the mask and blew it out again, the mask getting unpleasantly damp in the process. I didn't usually have time to attend operations on my patients but this was something special and good old Fred had said he would take surgery for me. Mr Ranjet Singh and his house surgeon were scrubbing up in the side-room; snatches of their conversation drifted through.

'How is old Mr Drayson doing? Tube draining all right?'

'Yes, sir, fluid's much clearer now and his temperature's settling, should be able to take it out soon.'

'Fine.'

The anaesthetic apparatus hissed and clicked in time with the patient's respirations; the anaesthetist, head bowed over her, occasionally glanced sideways at the dials and made slight adjustments to the flow of gas. The minutes ticked by on the wall clock; if anything, I was feeling more stifled now despite the fans – I wasn't stripped down to pyjamas under my gown like the operators.

I looked at the girl on the table, her face gripped by the mask, her slim figure almost completely covered by green sterile sheets. 'Theatre' was a good word – there was something unreal, yet poignantly dramatic about her role as an inert mummy-like figure there, the heroine of the play being enacted. In real life she was a beautiful Anglo-Indian girl, tall, quiet-mannered and singularly uncomplaining. It seemed a crude violation of her person that she was to be subjected to the surgeon's knife. . .

To be honest, I was concerned about myself as well. I'd called MacFarlane, the senior surgeon, to see her as I had been uncertain of the diagnosis. It seemed to me that he wasn't all that sure either, which was very unusual. Yet he'd agreed with me, and so had Singh who actually had to do the operation. 'Low grade appendicitis it is,' MacFarlane had concluded at last, in his grating Scots voice.

But why had he asked Singh to do a 'laparotomy', an *exploratory* operation if he was sure? It hadn't been at all straightforward, this case, with a very unusual history. Oh yes, pain on the right side all right, on and off for days, but no temperature rises that I could catch, no real bowel upset and very little sickness.

Well, we'd soon know the answer – and that patch of olive-coloured skin in the middle of the clipped sheets would yield it. Whatever it was, I, as her home doctor, would bear the ultimate responsibility. The buck would stop with me. . .

They *were* taking an age preparing. They didn't seem to be in any hurry to get started. I thought back over the case again.

Mrs Enslicott, the girl's mother, an equally striking Indian lady, had met her husband in East Africa, when he had been in the Air Force. She had shown obvious relief when I decided to call in MacFarlane. I was relieved that I had too, for that night I had had a phone-call from Enslicott himself. Now a barrister of the Middle Temple, he was only at home at the weekends. I had heard of his reputation: although a junior in chambers, he was quite clearly building a reputation as an expert in medico-legal cases – in fact, just the sort of person *not* to have as father of one of your patients.

He was very self-controlled, pleasant but cooly insistent. Had I been able to arrive yet at a diagnosis? Had I considered calling for a second opinion? If so, he was quite prepared to bring down a London consultant, if I so wished. Finally, 'Of course, doctor, I have the greatest confidence in your judgement.' I took that to mean, 'And you'd better be right, or else. . .'

'OK, George?' Ranjet Singh looked enquiringly at the anaesthetist. He nodded. As the incision penetrated the abdominal cavity a stream of fluid, deeply stained with dark blood, flowed out, to be mopped up rapidly by the assistant. 'This is no appendix,' muttered Singh. He probed gently. 'A right ovarian cyst is bleeding – unusual not to give rise to more symptoms. Must have been oozing on and off for days, by the history; not a lot, but the blood is widespread.' He half-turned his face towards me. 'Didn't complain of any shoulder pain, did she?'

'Yes, she did, last night. But it wasn't much and I thought she was just stiff from lying in bed so long.'

'Might have thought the same myself,' he said generously. 'But, as you know, it's a referred pain from the diaphragm which is being irritated by the blood in the peritoneal cavity – a cardinal sign.'

He paused and gently examined the left ovary. 'This one seems healthy, thank goodness. Don't like taking out ovaries in a young woman.'

When he was peeling off his operating kit afterwards in the dressing-room he put his hand on my shoulder. 'That ovary had no further function right from the start of her trouble.'

As I drove home, I went over the whole affair in my mind. Had I let her down in *any* way? Everyone can make mistakes in diagnosis and MacFarlane had too. Had I been negligent? I'd visited her every day and got advice, and that ovary could not have been saved even by early diagnosis.

Fine – but would Enslicott the medico-legal sleuth be of

the same opinion. I rang him that night as he had requested, told him all the details and added that one remaining healthy ovary would normally be quite capable of enabling her to bear children. There was what I can only call, unfelicitously, a pregnant pause. Then Enslicott's imperturbable voice said, 'Thank you, doctor, for informing me so fully and frankly. Good-night.'

On the advice of Charles and Fred, I took the precaution of putting the Medical Defence Union in the picture, just in case. All they said was, 'Do nothing, doctor, but make sure your case notes are in good order', which did not exactly assuage my apprehensions. In my prayers that night I took the matter to a 'higher court', and felt a lot better.

My greatest concern was for Aileen Enslicott, but, like the healthy young person she was, she recovered in double-quick time. Absolutely nothing of a legal nature transpired for me until, after a short engagement to a nice young Wilverton lad, she was legally bethrothed and I was invited to the wedding. I had appreciated by then that legal expertise can cut both ways. Despite Enslicott's emotional involvement in his daughter's case, he had realized that there were no valid grounds for an action, and certainly none for upsetting his daughter without real cause.

A little over a year after her marriage, Aileen gave birth to a lovely little boy to carry on his grandfather's line if not his name. They called the baby 'Godolphus', which rapidly became 'Gaddy' or 'Gad' for short, because of his early propensity to wander about. As they added to their brood over the years I smiled at the thought that 'Gad' in the Bible signifies 'Behold, a troop cometh'. The choice of name seemed little short of prophetic. There was certainly no cause to worry about the functioning of that single ovary!

Perhaps the Enslicott affair was only remotely connected with Africa, but it was through Aileen's father that I became spectator at another – an affair that started in England, travelled to South Africa and back to England once again.

After the wedding of his daughter, and even more after my successful assistance at the delivery of his first grandchild, Enslicott and I began developing a friendship somewhat beyond the limits of the usual good relations between doctor and patient. One evening, when Elisabeth and I were having coffee with him and Mrs Enslicott, he said, 'Any time you are in London, and I have a case in the Law Courts, why don't you come along and hear it? He grinned. 'You might be able to give me some tips.'

'I doubt whether they'd be much use,' I replied, 'but I'd very much like to do that. The law fascinates me with its insistence on facts not fancy – we could do with more of that from patients sometimes!'

'Huh! You'd be surprised at what seems to convince some juries.' He sounded really disillusioned for a moment. 'But ring up my chambers if you do come up to town and you have the time to look in. They'll tell you if I'm in court.'

It was two months later that I had to go to London for a council meeting of the missionary society I had been with in Africa. I found myself leaving Charing Cross station to head down the Strand in the direction of the Law Courts, pleasantly anticipating an interesting hour or two listening to a case with Enslicott in action.

As I strode through the crowds I began to analyse my feelings. What a nasty instinct had taken possession of me at the prospect of seeing some fellow creature, in this case a medical colleague, subjected to the rigours of public inquisition. I was looking forward to ricocheting 'for' and 'against' like a tennis ball as I listened first to plaintiff's and then defendant's case, enjoying the fact that it wasn't *my* actions that were coming under the legal microscope. Actually, I had already found for the defence, irrespective of what evidence might be produced, because the defendant was one of my own old hospital teachers – now extremely venerable – whom I knew to be a man of impeccable skill and integrity. In my book he had already won his case, and had been given judgement with costs!

And it truly was a most unusual case. A wealthy South African businessman living in London, had been operated on by this former surgical teacher of mine for a suspected growth in the bladder. On opening up that organ, the surgeon had found what he saw and felt was an inoperable cancer, so he simply closed the wound again. On the insistence of the patient he told him exactly what he had found and advised him if he so wished, to sell up and return to South Africa, as his days were numbered.

On arrival in South Africa, unexpectedly improved, the patient had seen another surgeon who had first cystoscoped him – this involved passing a sort of periscope through the urinary passage and viewing the interior. The surgeon decided that the growth looked operable, so he went ahead and removed a tumour which, on pathological examination, turned out to be non-malignant. Thirsting for retribution, if not hard cash, the patient had returned and sued my erstwhile teacher for damages for negligence.

When I arrived, unfortunately, Enslicott had already made his defence. This was based on the fact that you can see better with the naked eye into the bladder than through a cystoscope and that therefore the mistake was an error of judgement and not a case of negligence. He had called an 'expert witness' for his client – Enslicott himself had once told me that witnesses were either liars, d— liars or expert witnesses – and as I crept into the back of the court, the expert witness was already in the box for cross-examination, standing there cool and dignified.

Counsel for the plaintiff gathered his papers and his histrionic ability and, at the risk of severe damage to his larynx, delivered a long attack on the expert evidence, designed specifically to convince the jury of his client's case – namely that a cystoscopy had been essential. He ended with a question, his finger stabbing across the court at the witness.

'Now, sir, what have you to say in answer to that?'

The expert leaned forward, however, and said quietly but audibly, 'I did not hear all you said, would you repeat it please?'

The wretched Counsel stood for a moment in agonized unbelief, contracted visibly and in a monotone repeated his whole speech, all effect lost. 'Expert witnesses' evidently had their uses.

Both Counsels now summed up their case. The judge

instructed the jury and they left the box. They were gone a long time. To my great disappointment I had to leave too, before hearing the verdict, to catch my train. But I was confident that the defendant would win – particularly after the contribution of Enslicott's expert witness' – a cystoscope made no difference.

On my way home in the train, I opened the evening paper I had bought at the station. I could hardly believe my eyes. There was the verdict: my surgeon friend had gone down, to the tune of £6,000! And the decisive issue – he had not used a cystoscope! I felt that the law was indeed 'an ass' in this instance.

I leaned back in the corner seat and thought long and hard about the travesty of justice I had just witnessed. As I looked through the window at London's crowded suburbs flashing past, I couldn't help comparing them with the scattered dwellings of the Kenya hills, the complicated reasonings of the West with the homespun logic of a tribal court. Ideas ran on with the rhythm of the wheels. . .

I thought of the vacillating theological niceties of so many religious discussions on the radio, and contrasted them with one of the phrases old Kipkorir, our Kenyan carpenter, was fond of using: 'If a stone gets in your sandal, you can keep on walking, but it will lame you in the end. That is like the evil in the heart of a man.' Another carpenter had said even simpler yet more profound things some 2,000 years before: 'Why try to take a splinter from your brother's eye while you ignore the plank that is in your own?'

Jacobo, another friend from Kenya, in England to study public health at the Liverpool School of Tropical Medicine and Hygiene, had said to me only a few weeks earlier: 'I like your land of England and its green fertility, though I do not like your weather! I see the West has given many things to my country, some bad, some good. But the best of all is faith in Jesus Christ. But now the England that I see is like the ships I have seen in Mombasa. An engine drives these ships. Your engine is faith, but you have shut that engine off. The ship proceeds under its momentum for a time, but', and his voice filled with real dismay, 'soon the ship drifts on the rocks, for the steering-wheel of morality cannot guide without the engine. I pray to God that soon you start again the engine.'

5
That hideous strength

'Clang, clang, clang.' The house-lights dimmed and the roped square in the middle stood suddenly stark in the brilliance of the arc lamps. Within it, two pinked fleshed giants wheeled, crouched, and sprang, grappling at each other like two enormous and relatively hairless chimpanzees. The wrestling had begun on Wilverton Pier.

But what was a local practitioner doing there in the audience – accompanied by his brother-in-law, a well-known missionary from Central Africa? Surely this was a rather unlikely haunt for them?

It came about because Inspector Dai Jones of Wilverton Police is a most persuasive person.

'You're wanted on the phone.' Elisabeth called me in from the garden. I wasn't all that pleased, as it was my afternoon off and I was digging in the vegetable-patch.

A voice said, 'Docco, are you fit and flourishing?'

My irritation vanished as I recognized Dai's dulcet Welsh tones. We had played together in the Wilverton Rugby Club scrum for several years before I eventually acknowledged my age and hung up my boots. I had read recently in *The Wilverton Advertiser* that Sergeant Dai Jones was now 'Inspector'.

'Hullo, Inspector,' I replied. 'Nice to hear from you. What can I do for you?'

'Haven't forgotten your old pals then,' said Dai. 'That's just as well, man. I've got a job for you.' I wasn't sure what was coming next – our last 'job' had been when we were both involved in trying to solve a murder case. 'Feeling generous are you, docco?'

'Why, d'you want a contribution to the Police Widows' and Orphans' Fund?'

44

'No, no, nothing like that. Just some of your valuable time.' I could tell he was playing himself in with caution.

'Come on, Dai,' I joked, 'you know I charge heavily for anything outside the NHS. What is it you're after?'

'I can't promise you cash, just a free seat at the ring-side for a charity like. Wrestling on the pier – and a boys' club gets a percentage. We need a medical officer, the other doctor's gone off sick. Come on man, you'd love it – after all, you did plenty of wrestling yourself on the rugby field!'

I laughed. It might be fun. I hadn't seen wrestling since my school-days in London. 'You did your share too, Dai, don't forget. What about the time when you carried that French scrum-half off the field, ball and all?'

'Well, will you do it, docco?' We need someone next Wednesday.'

I thought quickly. Elisabeth's brother, John, and his wife were coming to visit us. He was a missionary, but a most unorthodox one who loved motor racing and sailing. I was pretty sure he'd be keen to come with me.

'OK, you're on.'

'Will you come at seven o'clock? You have to examine all the wrestlers before they fight, to see if they're fit. It's the rules, and if they get hurt you attend to them. But they don't get hurt often.'

'You must be joking – see if they're fit? Most of them could take you apart with one hand, Dai. I'll be there but I want two seats, please.'

John laughed when I told him. 'It's all just a great big con,' he said. 'I've read about it – they arrange who's going to win and the wrestling's phoney.'

'Well, we'll see,' I said.

I left John in his seat and went round to the changing room. The atmosphere was thick with human sweat and embrocation. An official introduced me to a fearsome array of young men of Herculean proportions. Before most of them I felt my six feet one inch only a pygmy stature. I read their names one by one off a list. 'Strangler Jake', 'The Black Assassin', 'Hercules Harris' and so it went on – names to strike terror into the souls of the faint-hearted.

45

There was no need and no time allowed for more than a cursory examination of hearts and reflexes as I went down the line with a stethoscope and a patella hammer. A sledge-hammer would have been more appropriate.

At the end a tall quiet man was standing. I thought I knew his face though now it was flabby and there were bags under his eyes. I read the programme: 'Mad Morgan, the Merioneth Mountain'. It couldn't be . . .

My mind raced back to the night before the Varsity Match in 1935, and the hotel in London's Piccadilly where the Cambridge Rugby fifteen, of whom I was one, were staying. I saw him now, standing there in the foyer in an evening suit: black curly hair, fine features and broad, bulging shoulders – Evans Morgan the boxer, British heavyweight champion. Surely it couldn't be this man? He was powerful still, but fat and obviously gone to seed. I couldn't resist trying to discover if he was the same person.

'Excuse me, are you "Evans Morgan the boxer"?' I asked.

The sombre face lit up and he smiled. His teeth were still in good shape though yellowed by tobacco. 'I am indeed,' he said.

'But you're from Swansea, not Merioneth, aren't you, unless I'm much mistaken?' I looked enquiringly up at him.

'Don't forget the appeal of alliteration, doctor. Truth is a secondary consideration in a wrestling title.' He had an educated voice, unmistakably Welsh in intonation. And there was a barely concealed Celtic sadness there when he said, 'You have a happy look to you, doctor. I would not have said your profession encouraged cheerfulness.'

'Well, this may sound odd, but I guess that being a Christian helps.' I tried not to sound sanctimonious.

He lifted his black eye-brows. 'I was raised in chapel myself, doctor. Sang in the choir with the best of them.'

I remembered how, even when he was in 'the fight game' he could get an audience anywhere with his guitar and tenor voice; in fact, his decline in boxing was due as much to playing in vaudeville and neglecting training, as anything else.

46

'I wish . . .' he began, but the warning ring-side bell clanged and I turned to go.

'Tell me,' I whispered quickly. 'Do you really compete or is it all arranged?'

'Ah, that would be telling, boyo, but I'll tell you one thing, this grip is genuine all right.'

He put out his huge hand and squeezed my neck just about the shoulder. My arm went dead and helpless. When he released me, my superspinatus muscle hurt like a toothache.

'Thank you. Thank you very much indeed for the demonstration,' I said with a wry smile.

'Sorry if I hurt you, doctor. It's nice to meet you. Perhaps I could give the old gospel another go, if it's not too late.'

'It's never too late,' I smiled, and left him.

My memory of the next hour or so is rather confused. Massive bodies were hurled to and fro in the ring, to land with excruciating violence on the floor, against the posts and ropes, or against one another. Arms and legs appeared to be on the point of total dislocation. Terrible injuries seemed inevitable, but the only work that came my way that night was when one of the 'giants' tripped, coming down the steps from the ring, and sprained his ankle.

The most entertaining event by far was a demonstration of self-defence by a sylph-like policewoman, and a large policeman dressed as her assailant. The damsel felled her unfortunate attacker with a series of kicks to the throat, arm-locks and throws, and eventually led him helpless from the ring to the ecstatic applause of the audience.

My friend Morgan lost his bout – whether by accident or design I shall never know. Having thrown his opponent from a considerable height on to his back, he turned his own on the recumbent figure and faced the crowd flexing his enormous biceps for all to admire. His opponent climbed surprisingly rapidly to his feet, seized Morgan from behind, tripped him and held his shoulders down to the boards the required number of seconds, thus gaining the victory by one fall to nothing.

Sadly, I don't know what happened to Morgan after that.

He seemed to disappear from the public eye, but I had cause some while later to be grateful for his instruction.

Inspector Jones's other extracurricular activity was helping to run the Wilverton Boys' Club and with true Welsh subtlety he inveigled me into getting involved in this too. His approach this time was rather more direct as the club was an entirely voluntary organization. He played again on my keenness for sport to get me to help examine the competitors in a club boxing tournament.

This was a much more serious medical commitment. Amateur boxing has very strict rules regarding the fitness of participants. I examined every boy in both teams thoroughly from top to toe. All went well until it was the turn of a hefty young fellow, the visiting heavyweight to be examined. Everything seemed satisfactory – until I tested his eyes. To my surprise he had a marked nystagmus – a sideways flicking of the eye, when he looked to the left.

'Have you been knocked out recently?' I asked.

The young man looked embarrassed – but he had to own up. He had concealed the fact that in a training bout a week earlier he had had a momentary concussion. Under no circumstances would I agree to his boxing in the competition that night.

He took it well – but his trainer didn't. I heard murmurs of 'nobbling' and 'dirty tricks' and decided that I had to deal with this quickly and firmly. 'I read the rules carefully before I came here,' I announced. 'This boy is unfit to box – and if my decision is questioned in any way, I shall report this matter to the Amateur Boxing Board. In any case I shall require his re-examination before he is allowed to recommence training. Is that clear?

The 'opposition' made no further protest, and – fortunately – the visiting team won by one bout.

Some weeks after this little episode I had an emergency call in the early evening. A woman's voice said, 'Doctor, could you come? I think Mrs Spendlove has injured herself in the kitchen.'

I was walking up the front path to the Spendloves' house

48

when I got wind of the true nature of the trouble. I could hear the crash of furniture, wails and loud shouting.

I opened the door and went straight into a scene of violence. Spendlove had always been fond of his pint at *The Crown* and evidently had had a few that night. Chairs were lying upturned all over the floor and Mrs Spendlove was crouching on the sofa shielding her head while he stood over her, his hand raised to strike.

'Stop that, you great bully!' I shouted and jumped forward.

'Who the hell do you think you are?' he bellowed, and took a swing at me with his right fist.

I parried the blow quite easily as he was half-drunk, and in the next split second I remembered Mad Morgan's agonizing shoulder-grip. With all the strength I could muster, I grabbed Spendlove above his left shoulder with my right hand. He yelled with pain and surprise, and then, with his arm hanging limply, to my astonishment, he collapsed on the sofa beside his wife and burst into tears. I let go of him and began examining Mrs Spendlove who was still sitting with a look of mute disbelief and fear on her face.

'He can't help it, doctor, when he's had a few. He'll be quiet now. Please don't hurt him any more.'

Nothing was further from my mind. In fact, I was rather bothered by the effect of what I had already done. Visions of a complaint for assault flashed before my mind.

To my amazement, Spendlove came to see me in the evening surgery two days later and apologized. We had a good chat and I found out that his two boys belonged to the club and that sometimes he looked in to watch the PT and boxing.

'Used to be quite handy myself,' he said, 'but I couldn't put one on you, doctor. You must have been a boxer yourself.'

I suggested he offered to train the boys at the club if the organizer would have him.

I went again just once to examine the boxers and Spendlove was there assisting as a second. 'Laying off the booze now,

49

doctor,' he whispered proudly, ''Ave to show them a good example.'

6
The jaws that bite

'It's only a prick, you'll hardly feel it.'

I smiled at Philip Hammond as he rolled up his sleeve to reveal a muscular arm. As sports master at Wilverton Grammar School he was in good physical shape. He was taking an expedition of boys from the fifth form to North Africa in the holidays and he needed immunization for typhoid.

'Doesn't worry me, doc,' he grinned, as I stuck the needle into his bulky shoulder muscle. 'Had lots of these in the army-y-y-.' I caught him just in time as he keeled over, ashen pale. He would have hit the floor with an awful bang. He was a huge man – the fall might not have damaged him much, but I wasn't so sure about the floor. I lowered him gently down.

'It's funny,' I thought. 'The bigger they are, the harder they fall. Probably wouldn't have bothered some slight little woman – they're the tough ones.'

He smacked his lips a few times, then opened his eyes and looked at me vacantly. His colour was coming back. He sat up and rubbed the top of his head ruefully.

'Sorry, doc, guess I've done it again.' In spite of his professed confidence he now admitted that at times the 'needle' upset him. I gave him a hand up and he heaved himself back on the chair. 'Haven't done that for a long time, honestly, doctor. Sorry,' he said again.

'That's OK – you are a bit of a weight though,' I replied.

From the postcard depicting a desert oasis, I guessed the school party was having the trip of a lifetime, but a week after they returned, Hammond was back in the surgery again. He had a swollen lower right jaw. 'Don't know if I've picked

51

up some sort of bug, doctor – this came up the day we got home.'

I tested his teeth and when I tapped a first molar, he winced.

'You've got a root abscess, I guess – job for a dentist,' I said. 'I'll start you off on penicillin tablets to contain the infection, but I'm afraid you'll probably lose that tooth.'

Next morning I had a call from Tomlinson, a dentist in the town. 'I've X-rayed Mr Hammond, and he has got an abscess. Would you come and give him gas for me?' We arranged for 12.15 the next day – the earliest I could manage.

I thought, as I put the mask on Philip Hammond's face, that he was looking a little apprehensive.

'Nothing to worry about. You won't feel a thing, just breathe away quietly.'

No sooner had the nitrous oxide and oxygen begun to work than Hammond started to squirm and jerk in his chair even though there was a broad strap around his waist to prevent his slipping down. However, he was quite unconscious and Tomlinson whipped out the tooth with great dexterity and plugged a swab on the gap where discharge was beginning to drain.

His technique was first class, but he'd barely got his finger out of Hammond's mouth before his jaws clamped shut and he began to thrash about with his arms and legs. Tomlinson did his best to hold his legs, but Hammond was a powerful man and he flung him off and dealt the tray holding the expensive dental equipment an almighty kick which scattered forceps, probes and other instruments around the room. Although he knew the patient was unaware of the chaos he was causing and was only in a state of unconscious excitement caused by the gas, Tomlinson himself seemed to lose all control and reason and shouted, 'Stop it, stop it!' As Hammond's flailing legs continued to threaten the surgery with imminent destruction, Tomlinson dealt him quite a lusty punch in the side.

Now it was *my* turn to shout to Tomlinson, 'Stop that for goodness' sake! Have you gone mad?'

52

He gesticulated wildly. 'Look at my surgery – he's wrecking it!'

Whether it was the effect of the shouting or the punch in the side or merely the anaesthetic wearing off, Hammond calmed down, his eyes opened and he leaned drunkenly forward to spit out blood and discharge and wadding into the little glass bowl with the stream of running water.

'Did I behave badly again?' He half-turned his head to me. I patted him on the shoulder and give him a glass of pink fluid to wash out his mouth. Tomlinson was forlornly gathering up his scattered equipment.

I wiped the sweat from Hammond's face and undid the strap. 'Come and sit in the waiting-room for a minute. Then I'll take you home. I expect you could do with a lift.' He didn't live far from me.

I went back into the surgery. I was feeling both angry and worried. Tomlinson looked at me abashed. 'Sorry, old boy – lost my head for a moment.'

I felt sorry for *him*, but what he'd done was both unprofessional and unforgiveable, even though it may have arrested Hammond's mayhem. Such a thing had never happened before in all my experience and it wasn't likely ever to happen again, yet something had to be said.

'Don't ever do a thing like that again, will you, no matter *what* a patient does. If you ever lose control and I'm giving the anaesthetic – it'll be the last one you get from me. We'll be lucky if he doesn't sue us for assault! He'd be quite justified in doing so.'

He hung his head. 'Don't know what possessed me – but all this stuff is brand new, you see. I couldn't bear to see it wrecked.' He smiled miserably.

'Well, never mind, let's hope Hammond was still too flat out to know what was happening,' I said as I left the surgery.

In my heart, I knew I was partly to blame. For all his robust appearance, it was obvious that Hammond was a tense person and injections and anaesthetics were too much for him to cope with. I should have foreseen trouble.

Hammond sat quietly in the car until we were half-way home. I saw through the corner of my eye that he was quietly

53

rubbing his left ribs. I knew he was far too tough to have suffered any real harm from that punch. He half-turned towards me.

'What was I really doing, doctor? I guess I needed thumping.' So he knew!

'Let's forget it,' I said; I fervently hoped he would – and he did.

I sat by the fire that evening and brooded over dental battles of the past.

There was the patient in the East End where I worked during the London blitz. It was in the out-patients' department of a small mission hospital, and we housemen did lots of unusual things including dental extractions.

This particular chap had a mouth full of huge, decayed teeth. He was the mildest of men. Week after week he came, and each time we extracted more and more of his teeth. And every time he fought like a tiger, threatening us (through his mask) in his half-conscious state with awful things – and in the most colourful language. After each session he was consumed with agonized remorse and appeared to go away a broken man. Next time, however, the pantomime was repeated in every detail. By the end of six weeks we were feeling years older, the other houseman and I.

Finally, resplendent with a shining new set of choppers, he presented us with an almost unobtainable box of chocolates which must have used up months of his sweet rations. 'Ain't eatin' any more of these,' he said. Unfortunately, it was a bit late in the day for such a commendable resolution!

Then there was the second officer with toothache on board the ship taking Elisabeth and me to Africa in 1943. The ship's doctor discovered I could extract teeth. I whipped out the officer's tooth for him but his way of showing his gratitude was to duck me unmercifully in the swimming pool during the crossing-the-line ceremonies.

In Africa itself, I'd been stopped on one occasion on safari by a tribal warrior who demanded that I remove an offending molar from his formidable jaw.

No anaesthetic was available in the bush – but he belonged to a tough race. He sat on the ground and, though sweat poured from his handsome face, he never uttered a sound. After a ten-minute struggle, when the forceps were almost dropping from my nerveless hand, out came the tooth *and* the one next to it – jerked out by the crown of the first, and the power of my strong right arm. Fortunately for me, the second tooth had a large hole in it as well, so I was able to point out to the warrior that he had had two for the price of one.

As I saw the young man departing, armed again with spear and club, I was grateful for that hole in the second tooth. Africans set great store by their teeth and the unintentional removal of a good one might have had dire consequences for me.

I hoped most fervently that Philip Hammond's remaining teeth would see him through for many years – or at least until after my retirement from any connection with human jaws. So far I had avoided harm, but one day I felt a pair of jaws might well snap shut on me.

7

Booze and Billy Graham

The card said: 'Mrs Esther J Asburton'. I knew the surname – Mickey Asburton was a pillar of Wilverton Rugby Club. In my playing days, I had often met him after matches when I was consuming my modest ginger-beer in the bar of the local with the teams. He was a jolly, hail-fellow-well-met sort of chap and a keen supporter. True, as the manager of the small but flourishing local industry, 'Sussex Sports, Makers of Games Equipment', he had a vested interest. The firm supplied the club with rugby balls and kit, but the main item of their enterprise was the renowned 'Wilverton Willows', nationally-famed cricket bats, made from the trees which grew in the weald beyond the Downs.

A quiet knock came on the surgery door and an attractive lady walked in. 'Forty-five', I calculated quickly from the date of birth shown on the bottom of the record-card. Dark-haired and small-featured, she had a trim figure which belied the fact that she had had four children, their births being almost the only items recorded in the envelope.

'Good morning, Mrs Asburton, please sit down.' I shook hands – a practice I've found seems to put patients more at ease. 'I don't think we've met before, have we, though I do know your husband. I hope he's well. Now, what have you come to see me about?'

'Yes, he's well thank you, doctor.' I sensed a tiny suggestion of doubt in her voice. 'I feel fine. It's almost an imposition, coming to see you at all about such a small matter, but I wondered whether you could help me with a few tablets. I'm not sleeping at all well.'

A look of unutterable weariness came into her grey eyes. It had probably been quite an effort to persuade herself to come to the doctor at all. I resisted the temptation simply to do what she asked and give her a prescription for a sedative. It's too easy, in the rush of a busy surgery, to dish out something; antacids for indigestion, linctus for coughs, laxatives for constipation, antibiotics for infections – just like a booking clerk issuing tickets for a journey to the chemist's shop down the road. Charles's words, 'Examine the patient', filtered through my tired brain. I *was* tired – entirely my own fault. I'd had a long session the night before at a meeting organized by our vicar, Algernon Greenfield, to form a committee, and it had been a bit much at the end of a hard day.

'Have you always slept well before?' I made myself ask.

'Yes, of course, except when the children were babies. They got me up a bit,' she added a little wistfully.

I thought, 'I hope Mickey got up sometimes too.'

'Any reason for your not sleeping now? Any tummy trouble, waterworks trouble, cramp? Do you still have periods? Perhaps she was getting menopausal sweats which disturbed her sleep.

'No, no trouble anywhere.'

'Well, we'd better give you the once-over.'

I stood up, swinging my stethoscope. There was nothing abnormal in chest, heart, colour of eyes, abdomen or blood pressure. I sat down again and looked at her. 'Is there anything on your mind?'

I half-expected it; her eyes fell, two tears welled out and rolled down her cheeks. She quickly opened her bag and dabbed at them with a handkerchief.

'Doctor, I hate saying this, but – I'm afraid my husband is becoming an alcoholic. I don't mean simply that he drinks regularly. After all, we've been used to wine with meals and he often had a whisky before going to bed, if he'd had a bad day. And I don't mean he comes home drunk every night. But I *know* things aren't right. He's unbearable in the mornings but much nicer if I meet him for lunch in town. His secretary is always ringing up about work he's forgotten, and he's getting through bottles and bottles of whisky. He puts them out in the rubbish-bin himself, but I know. He spends a lot of time in the private bar of the local too. It

57

worries me so much, especially as he has so much driving to do for the business.

'I'm sure this is why I can't sleep. I didn't come about him, but I'm glad I told you. Please, can anything be done for Mickey?'

Though she'd only just met me, she'd called her husband by his Christian name in her concern, without even noticing.

'Yes, it can, but – it's not that simple. He must *want* help. He must admit he needs it, and that'll be hard for him to face. If he really wanted something done about it, we could set about treatment. Get the alcohol out of his system, see what damage it may have done, build him up and perhaps give him something that will make any drink disgusting to him. But he must have the incentive to begin and keep on with the treatment. If he is a genuine alcoholic, it will mean him being on the water-wagon for life. Would he come and see me?'

'Oh, I'm sure he wouldn't. He'd probably be angry with me for talking to you about him. Couldn't you perhaps come and see him like a friend and then talk to him?'

'I don't think that would work. It would put it all on the wrong footing. The initiative must come from him. I suggest you put it to him – pick your opportunity and, if he's willing, I'll do my best to help.'

I wasn't surprised as the days passed and I heard nothing from the Asburtons. It's a sad fact that alcoholics sometimes need to get to the end of their resources of self-deception and their ability to cope before they agree to seek help. I had to put Mrs Asburton's sad face out of my thoughts. I hadn't given her sleeping tablets, as she had seemed comforted by just sharing her problem.

It was a few days later that I ran into old Blenkinsop. I was preoccupied at the time. I had just visited a girl with glandular fever and she wasn't clearing up as I had hoped. 'Ran into' was almost literally true as I hurried out of the gate and almost landed on top of him as he passed. My side-step would have done credit to a top-class stand-off half.

'Sorry, Mr Blenkinsop, I . . .'

Before I could finish, he interrupted, 'Oh doctor, I'm so glad I met you, that will save a visit. First though, how is my little Sarah?'

A vision flashed through my mind of a husky maiden, now a five-foot-eight teenager, the terror of the lacrosse team. Blenkinsop was a benign little man, a good four inches shorter. He and his wife had been joint heads of the little school where our daughter Sarah had started her education in Wilverton.

'She's fine, Mr Blenkinsop. Hopes to go to university next year. Kind of you to remember her.'

'So glad, so glad. Actually it was another matter I wanted to see you about. I have something to give you.' He fished in his inside jacket-pocket, produced a well-worn wallet and from it drew a cheque which he handed to me. It was for fifty pounds and in my name.

'What is this for?' I asked, out of my depth, but pleased at this sudden unexpected windfall.

'Well, doctor,' he seemed shy all of a sudden, 'we were so impressed, my wife and I, with the campaign of Dr Billy Graham in London, that when we heard there had been a film made of it, we thought that it would be a good idea to get it for a cinema in Wilverton. This is a contribution to help defray some of the initial expenses. We're not really *au fait* with the procedures involved, so we thought perhaps you would be able to get a committee together to organise it.'

I was a little puzzled as to why they should think a GP would know any more about such matters than themselves – or indeed, would have the time to do this – but all I said was, 'What a good idea and very generous of you. Yes, I'll deal with it.' I didn't tell them that they weren't first with the idea – Algernon's meeting the week before had been about just that, and I had, together with my partner Charles, already agreed to help. This gift did seem like a confirmation of Algernon's scheme.

After this, money simply streamed in from all sides and we booked the local cinema for a whole week. We asked an old friend, part-evangelist, part-farmer and a former officer in the Coldstream Guards, to come and follow up the showing each night with a few well-chosen words. He had once, years before, knocked all the stuffing out of the Cambridge Rugby XV in my college rooms with his stories of the Christian's life. We thought he had the right approach to appeal to all sections of our community.

The Reverend Algernon Greenfield is a dangerous man to work with. He is apt to come up with the weirdest schemes. On this particular occasion, his voice over the phone said, 'Andy, would you feel like coming with me on a pub-crawl?' Immediately I had visions of headlines in *The Wilverton Advertiser*; 'Local vicar and doctor involved in drunken brawl.'

'You're doing what?' I gasped.

'Thought that would have you guessing,' he laughed. 'I'm going round all the pubs in the parish with invitations for the Billy Graham film. Will you join me? I may need protection.'

Here was a challenge I couldn't resist. 'OK, I'll come.'

'Meet me outside *The Carpenter's Arms* at nine, it should be full then.' He rang off.

We had a great time on our 'tour'. Algie knew all the publicans in Wilverton. He would ask permission, then he or I would say our piece and give out invitations to the astonished customers propping up the bars. Algernon's formula for refusing the generous libations offered everywhere was to say, 'Thanks all the same but we've got to go round the lot. Just imagine what state we'd be in at the end if we accepted!'

Number four on his list was *The Door in the Wall*, a coaching inn dating back to the early eighteenth century. It had a log fire burning in an ingle-nook fireplace, and cosy subdued lighting. In a corner I spotted Mickey Asburton with some of my old rugby pals. He didn't seem too enthusiastic in returning my wave.

Life had to go on, even though the 'film week' was looming large on the horizon. I got a lot of leisure exercise in the garden under Elisabeth's expert direction, but now, as the nights were drawing in, there wasn't so much normal digging and other hard labour, so we thought we'd build a pond and rockery. But where to get stone for the rockery?

My old friend Joe Butterworth, 'Buttercup Joe' as he was known locally, knew everybody and everything in Wilverton. 'Try Farmer Jenkins, up your road,' he advised me. 'He's pulling down an old wall in his yard. He might let you have some stones cheap too, if you get on his right side.'

Jenkins was as unpredictable as Algernon, but in a different way. He was constantly at war with neighbouring farmers over his boundaries, and yet he could be quite generous in letting scout troops camp on his land free. I knew this because I sometimes had to attend to the casualties from some of their more dangerous enterprises, like swinging over chasms on ropes.

'Yes, you can have as much stone as you can take,' he said.

'How much will it cost?' I asked, following Elisabeth's advice to 'get a price first'.

'Oh, I won't overcharge you,' was all I could get out of him. 'But you'll have to break it out and cart it yourself.'

Peter and Barney were home for half-term, and Sarah was always ready to muck in with the boys, so they all came to help. We worked with a will until by the end of the afternoon we had carted home all we wanted in a big wheelbarrow.

'How much do I owe you, Mr Jenkins?'

'What are they charging over at quarry?' he quizzed me under his shaggy eyebrows.

'Fifteen pounds a ton,' I answered. I knew because I had enquired. I thought, 'Surely he won't have the nerve to charge us the quarry price when we've done all the work!'

'How much do you think you've got?'

'About three tons,' I said thinking, 'I simply can't afford forty-five pounds.'

'Well, make me an offer.'

I could see he was testing me. He knew I was a Christian. If I named too low a figure, he would consider me stingy, but I couldn't afford a lot.

'No, you give me a price.' I wasn't going to be taken for a ride.

'All right,' he relented. 'You send five pounds to Cancer Relief and we'll call it a day.'

'Thanks, Mr Jenkins,' I said, with an inaudible but heart-felt sigh of relief. Inside I was saying, 'Sorry for thinking you were a hard old blighter!'

'Would you have a look at one of these?' I gave him one of our Billy Graham leaflets.

'What's this? Billy Graham? Religion – no thanks!'

'It's a good film,' I said.

'Doubt I've got the time,' was all he'd say.

There was a good turn-out for the film, a full house every night. I'd had my reservations too when Billy Graham had first come to Britain, thinking that this hotted-up American mass-evangelism would be a nine days' wonder. But it hadn't been. Elisabeth and I went to hear Dr Graham ourselves. Yes, he *was* simplistic, there was a lot he *didn't* say, but it was what he *did* say that mattered. We later found that our African mission was getting recruits from men and women who had become Christians at the campaign and now felt that God wanted them to spend their lives telling other people the good news about a new life with Jesus Christ.

Our Coldstream Guard officer spoke in exactly the right way at each showing of the film. I was amazed when I saw Asburton and his wife there twice during the week, and on the last night, just as the curtain went up I spotted Jenkins creeping in at the back. I took the receipt from the Cancer Research Fund to give him, to show good faith.

'How did you like the film?'

'Good film, I'll grant you. What I didn't like was that speaker bloke afterwards. Said all our good deeds were just so many "filthy rags" as far as God was concerned, and didn't count for anything. Rot, he was talking, and cheek I call it, saying we don't get any credit for the good we do.'

'He didn't make it up himself, Mr Jenkins, here it is,' I said, showing him a verse from the book of Isaiah in my pocket Bible. Luckily, it was one of the verses I always found easy to remember.

'You mean it's in the Bible? Well!' He walked away

muttering for, like most good countrymen, he had a built-in reverence for scripture.

The following week both the Asburtons came to the surgery together. Mickey Asburton opened the batting.

'I want to do that course you talked to Esther about. I've got the incentive now, doc.' I looked at his wife. Her eyes were very bright.

We fixed up for Mickey to go to a drying-out place in Kent, what would now be called a 'detoxification centre'. He would have liver tests and general assessment, be given sedatives, if necessary, while he had a period of withdrawal from all alcohol, massive doses of vitamins and anything else that would rebuild his health and send him out a fit man.

Mickey and Esther Asburton joined Algernon's church. It became an annual pilgrimage for Algernon, Mickey and me to go to Twickenham together for the Oxford and Cambridge rugby match. We would celebrate in tea if the 'right' side won – that is, Cambridge!

Much later I heard that Mickey Asburton had chartered a special coach to take any of his firm's employees who wanted to go to one of the meetings at the next Billy Graham campaign in London. The bus was full.

8

Farewell the tranquil mind

Out of the clear, blue sky over Wilverton – and for once the town was topping the sunshine league – a cloud, as it were, appeared, at first 'no bigger than a man's hand'. But unlike the one that came in answer to the prophet Elijah's prayer in the Bible, heralding the relief of Israel from drought, this one was a harbinger of disaster. It made no headlines in the local press, but it was more threatening to our practice than a cut in the capitation payment for patients, more ominous than the appointment of a new Minister of Health.

The truth was that our receptionist, Miss Spencer, was contemplating retirement.

'Are you aware, doctor,' she said to Charles, who heads the practice, at the end of morning surgery when the last patient had left, 'that I am now past sixty-five? I will have to think seriously about retiring.'

As he informed us, Charles's first instinct after he had recovered from the initial shock of the approach of the unthinkable was to laugh it off as a momentary aberration of mind on her part. But he saw the earnest look in the grey eyes behind Miss Spencer's spectacles, and paused. Shakily he began, 'My dear Miss Spencer . . .' In over fifty years no one in the practice had presumed to use her Christian name. 'This is a heavy blow. Please can you give us time to consider?' She graciously assented.

Before us lay a prospect too grim for contemplation.

We might be left to the tender mercies of Mrs Badger, who, faithful though she was, was never so happy as when she stood, on Miss Spencer's afternoon off, alone and defiant like the boy on the burning deck, with chaos all around her in the waiting-room – a state of affairs capable of bringing on a severe attack of temporary nervous instability in the doctors taking surgery. The impending loss of the tranquillity always surrounding Miss Spencer weighed heavily upon all our minds. For half a century her office had seemed like the still centre of the cyclone, with patients, telephone calls, prescription demands and correspondence whirling about her unruffled person with bemusing rapidity.

Despite our delaying tactics, the 'cloud' grew steadily bigger as the days went by until, two months later, her departure became almost a *fait accompli*.

Happily for us, Miss Spencer, with her customary forethought on our behalf, had seen the yawning gap which her departure would leave in the organization. She had kept her trump card up her sleeve, delaying the dramatic dénouement of producing it until she was absolutely sure of its validity. Now she quietly presented it.

'May I suggest,' she murmured at the practice meeting Charles had called to consider the gravity of our situation, 'Mrs Banbury as my successor?'

The lady in question was apparently a perfect paragon, a person of many parts, as occasion required. Although at present the assistant secretary of a nearby girls' school, she was equally capable, at the drop of a hat, of taking over as assistant matron or of acting as confidante in teenage affairs of the heart. Altogether a pearl of great price in any doctor's surgery – provided, of course, the price wasn't too great.

'How do we know she would be available?' asked Fred.

Miss Spencer smiled a comfortable, knowing smile. 'I happen to have heard that the school is having to reduce its staff this term and so Mrs Banbury's services will no longer be required.'

When we phoned to ask the headmistress whether she could recommend Mrs Banbury, as we were thinking of inviting her to join our staff, her enthusiasm was inspiring.

'You're lucky to get in first,' she said. 'We're very sorry to lose her, she's been a real asset to the school.'

We couldn't ask for more than that, so we requested Mrs Banbury to come for an interview. She appeared a calm and charming person and the terms were reasonable. She was engaged. She worked with Miss Spencer for two weeks to learn the ropes. We didn't want a dragon at the desk, but at times we needed an inoffensive line of defence. Not every patient is a shining example of sweet reason, nor is every doctor for that matter – so a buffer state sometimes protects both. Mrs Banbury's reactions augured well for the future. When Miss Spencer's notice ran out, she took over.

Her typing was excellent though lacking the originality we had become accustomed to with Miss Spencer. Her approach was different; keeping her school charges in order had indeed inserted some iron into her soul. She was more incisive than her predecessor and she gave the patients less rope, but perhaps she meant to make a no-nonsense impression at the start and ease up later. We felt that if she had handled a girls' school of 200, a mere 7,000 patients should be child's play.

Before long, however, Mrs Banbury's mettle was put to the test. If I'd been able to, I would have spared her early contact with Seamus O'Flaherty. She filled in the details of her first encounter to me later. He had appeared at morning surgery evidently spoiling for a fight. On being told that, as he had made no appointment, he would have to wait until the end of surgery to see me, he had leant across the reception desk, seized the appointments book, twisted it round and stabbed a grubby finger on a blank space.

'And wot about dis den? Sure an' Oi'm not prepared to wait for de docthor jist to please yerself!'

'That space is left for the doctor to catch up on time overspent on patients. Will you kindly leave my book alone, Mr O'Flaherty?'

She became aware that the outlook was becoming distinctly ugly so she called me on the internal phone. I strode quickly into the surgery.

'If you're not out of here in twenty seconds, Mr O'Flaherty, I'll call the police.'

Surprisingly he left the surgery without a word. I was relieved as I was uncertain what the police would have done had they been called, but it had seemed the only thing to do at the time.

It was an even bigger surprise when he meekly made an

appointment later, for the next day, and came without any fuss. His symptoms suggested bronchitis and he was a heavy smoker. When he came to pull up his shirt for me to examine him, I was intrigued with the intricate pattern of flags and anchors with which his chest was adorned, but even more by the letters ALI over the right and nestling in the main motif. As I finished writing his prescription and he was tucking in his shirt, I inquired, 'Had an Arab friend once, did you, Mr O'Flaherty?' indicating the right side of his chest with my ballpoint.

If his rugged complexion had been capable of it, I'd swear he blushed.

'Well, docthor, I confess it was loike dis. I was havin' me wife's name inscribed on me chest, to surproise her, ye understand, when we was put in to Port Said on our way home. De old tatooist feller was jist halfway t'rough when de mate he comes bustin' in sayin' de boat was leavin', so I upps and runs for it. Niver got it finished, see? Her name was Alice,' he concluded rather lamely.

I thought that all was forgiven and forgotten, but I had misjudged O'Flaherty. He must have made a speedy recovery, for he did not revisit the surgery – at least, not in daylight hours.

Three weeks later I went in early on a Monday morning to make a good start. I found Mrs Banbury in a state bordering on acute distress. She had arrived even earlier, anticipating the Monday morning rush of patients who had saved up their ailments all weekend, to find the door already open. She had hurried to the back door which she found open too, and peering out, she had caught a fleeting glimpse of a man climbing over the back fence to make good his escape.

The surgery was in a state of chaos; drawers pulled out, contents of cupboards scattered over the floors and our typewriter gone. Curiously, she had also found a half-empty coffee-cup by my examination couch and the wall-heater above full on. It suggested that the intruder had treated himself to a cup of our coffee, lain down to relax in comfort on the couch and fallen asleep, only to awake just in time to avoid a confrontation with Mrs Banbury.

She had already called the police and they arrived a minute or two after me. When Charles joined the party, we were all solemnly finger-printed by a lugubrious plain-clothes detective and then the rooms were searched for further and hopefully alien prints. The drawer where we kept the petty cash had been rifled, and they found some on that. The discovery almost brought a momentary smile to the detective's countenance.

Inspector Dai Jones informed us later that 'they were doing their best and following up all leads', but the weeks went by without any arrest being made. Our major concern was that the situation should not recur – it is quite a strain coping with patients whilst trying to get the place back to rights. The only thing we needed was our typewriter; all dangerous drugs were kept to a minimum and were well locked up.

It was all due to the keenness of a new young constable back on the beat that the malefactor was eventually 'nabbed'. On his rounds on the other side of Wilverton late one night, he noticed an invalid car parked down an ill-lit side-street. There were two occupants. As he approached, one of them leapt out and 'scarpered'. The other got himself caught in the front seat behind the steering-wheel. The policeman found a sack in the back where the wheelchair should have been for a genuine invalid and, inside it, a tidy haul of drugs and surgery gear from another practice that side of the town. The man in the driving seat was – O'Flaherty.

At his flat they found our typewriter under the bed. It seemed that success in burgling our surgery had emboldened him to have another go. The invalid car, stolen for the occasion, would have provided a nice camouflage and transport for the swag, but for the sharp eyes of the bobby. Maybe starting with us had simply been O'Flaherty's way of getting his own back.

'We'd better go in for some burglar-proofing,' said Charles. 'Even though your friend's out of circulation, we don't want it giving other people ideas.'

I wondered if Pinkerton, another of our patients, might tighten up the surgery's security for us. He was a useful odd-job man and had put new locks on my house. 'Shall I pop round and see him?'

I found that Pinkerton himself was out but his wife, a cheerful, rosy-cheeked lady, asked me to come in and she would take down the details. I sat on a chair in the living-room. The atmosphere was steamy and redolent of soap-powder. Mrs Pinkerton pulled aside the 'whiter-than-white' washing from the high fireguard to let me see the fire, then she took down the particulars in a notebook. I was somewhat distracted by three or four small children – also very clean – who sat on the floor throughout the interview and fixed me with the unembarrassed, unwinking gaze of the very young.

The Pinkertons were frequent 'customers' of the practice, none more so than Mrs Pinkerton herself. She was not ill, just prolific. She had had seven children, all girls, and she looked about twenty-three, which, of course, short of a miracle, would have been legally impossible. In fact, she was thirty-two.

'We want Chubb locks on the outside doors and safety catches on the windows.' She took it all down.

When Pinkerton's estimate arrived it was reasonable and he soon had the work completed. 'Wife's in to see you tomorrow,' he told me as he packed up his tools.

'Not ill, I hope.'

'No, the usual,' he said with a suspicion of a smirk.

'Not . . .?'

'Yes, doctor, you see we do want a boy to complete the family.'

The baby, when it came six months later, was a bouncing – *girl*. Meanwhile, O'Flaherty and his accomplice, to our amazement, had been given bail on the first hearing, and we were annoyed to learn that we could not have our typewriter back as it was still wanted for evidence.

Despite his belligerency and burglarious propensities, we couldn't help liking O'Flaherty. He could turn on the Irish blarney and charm at the drop of a hat. However, when someone has entered your surgery, stolen your possessions and deliberately left havoc in his wake, there is inevitably a certain loss of the mutual trust necessary for a good doctor-patient relationship. So we felt, without any undue display of vindictiveness, that it was time he sought fresh woods and pastures new in the shape of another practice, and we took him off our list, and his wife with him.

It takes fourteen days for this to become effective. Maybe it was poetic justice or maybe just an example of Irish humour that, on the thirteenth day, O'Flaherty should choose to ask for a night call for his wife.

'And sorry it is I am to be botherin' ye, docthor, but I'm thinking 'tis an appendicitis that's she's got.'

Though I hardly had the sleep out of eyes when I examined her. I was quite certain that whatever she had it was *not* an appendicitis. A much more likely explanation was the tinned pilchards and toasted cheese supper that she had had. His thanks as I left were profuse.

O'Flaherty was duly tried and got six months and we got back our typewriter. Apparently there was a good deal more on his slate than just these two offences. His friend simply got a heavy fine and probation.

It seemed an incongruous thing to do but I sent O'Flaherty a letter in Lewes Prison and enclosed copies of some Bible reading notes. There was a short passage to read for each day, plus some straightforward explanatory comments. The copies I sent would last for the duration of his stay. I got no acknowledgement.

Following O'Flaherty's departure from the scene, the practice enjoyed a season of relative calm and Mrs Banbury had a chance to find her feet. I took the opportunity of visiting Miss Spencer in her home in the village of Brendon. I walked down the little drive to the house past clumps of red dogwood, yellow blossoms of winter jasmine and inhaled the scent of the early flowerets of a daphne bush. I felt there was plenty to occupy her here in her retirement, with her brother to help with the heavier work.

To my surprise I found her in bed. Her room looked out through a latticed window on the front garden and over the wall to the quiet Sussex valley beyond. Sitting up in bed she could see most of it.

'Just a troublesome bit of backache,' she said, but her appearance belied it. On the phone her own doctor told us that there was evidence of malignant secondary growths in her spine and elsewhere. The outlook was hopeless.

She lasted just over a month. We joined the crowds of old patients, former Sunday school pupils and relatives at her funeral.

'Of course, I realize that the primary growth must have been present before she retired,' said Charles afterwards. 'But my feeling is that when the book of her life in the practice was closed, it was too much for her to start another.

A year later, emotions of dismay, wonderment and mirth fought for supremacy in me when Mrs Pinkerton reappeared in the surgery. She had an obstinate triumphant look as she said, 'We do want a boy, doctor.' But, after a faultless pregnancy, she had twins – both girls. When we made the diagnosis, early on, we did hope that they would be dissimilar and that at least one would be a boy, but it was not to be.

'Be content,' we told her, but she still had that look of obstinacy. Back she came six months later with the light of battle in her eye. In contrast with the others, this was a bad pregnancy: morning sickness, later on toxaemia and later still depression, but she was delivered, with little more difficulty than usual, of a – boy! At last!

'Now, you've got your full team, ten girls and a boy, we don't want to see you again!' I told her at the post-natal check-up. She nodded. The piles of washing were larger than ever when I visited the family for the usual bouts of children's ailments.

'Don't tell me, I can't bear it!' I cried in disbelief when Mrs Pinkerton came in, obviously blooming, and equally obviously once again expecting. This, her eleventh pregnancy, reverted to the uneventful norm, and at the end there was a little Tony to join his brother Len in friendly rivalry for their sisters' attention.

'I really have finished doctor,' she said the next time I called. 'No more, *definitely*.' And she kept her word. . . .

The following summer, Elisabeth and I were going to

church when I stopped the car suddenly. On the zebra crossing ahead was a line of ten girls in ascending sizes. The
two tallest were pushing a pram and a push-chair. 'The
Pinkertons' team, with one reserve,' I pointed. 'On their way
to Sunday school.'

The man who entered the surgery had dark, curly hair, going
grey; he was quieter and showed no aggression, but there
was no mistaking O'Flaherty.

'It's meself, docthor', he announced. 'Oive lost even de
other half of me Alice now – ran away with me mate while
I was in gaol, and 'tis married dey are. Oi'm back at last in
me old haunts and de Catholic Fathers have given me a room
in deir hostel. Found me a job on de Municipal as well. A
refuse collector Oi am. Would ye be takin' me back on yer
list, docthor? Oi promise t'will only be by day Oi visits ye.'
His blue eyes twinkled.

'OK, Mr O'Flaherty, it's a deal.'

He grinned and thanked me. On the way out he said,
serious for once, 'Still readin' dem little books ye sent me,
docthor. Oi buy 'em meself, from de bookshop. Keep me
on de straight and narrow dey do.'

Whenever I passed the corporation dust-cart, I kept my
eyes skinned. Sure enough, more often than not, I got a
cheery wave from one man carrying a bin.

9

The house
that Jack built

Poor Johnny Taggerty, he seemed right off form today. First
he'd thrown his breakfast on the floor; now he just sat and
glowered at me and tried to push me away when I wanted
to examine him. He wouldn't even answer when I spoke.
It's hard when you're five and your brother and sister are
out playing in the garden and you can't be. Mercifully for
them, they were a healthy pair and showed none of the signs
of Johnny's trouble, though they could have done. He had
cystic fibrosis.

Physically he looked under-sized though mentally he was
quite up to scratch. Usually we got on very well. He still
loved the old nursery rhymes that I remembered from my
childhood. But, woe betide me if I got anything wrong or
left a word out when I recited them to him. He would pull
me up in a trice. His favourite was the one about the cow
with a crumpled horn which ends with 'the malt that lay in
the house that Jack built'. I would draw him little pin-men
and animals, which were about the limit of my artistic skill,
to supplement the tale. The pads supplied by a pharmaceut-
ical firm came in handy for this – the advertisements for their
latest anti-depressive tablet at the bottom of each page meant
nothing to Johnny.

But he couldn't have cared less about anything today. As
I suspected, when I did manage to examine his chest, he had
obviously got a fresh lung infection and we would have to
step up the dose of the antibiotic which he took as a routine
precaution. It would take several days for him to recover the
ground he had lost. Research into this congenital disease
might offer hope in time for improving the quality and length
of life of sufferers, but it looked as if it would come too late
for Johnny. He would never build a house like 'Jack'.

As I drove home for lunch, I hummed that favourite rhyme that he hadn't wanted today . . . 'the house that Jack built', 'that Jack built – that Jack built' – the wórds kept repeating in my head. Of course! That's what *we* ought to do – build a house. Johnny Taggerty was forgotten. . .

We'd been thinking the question over for weeks, Elisabeth and I. The trouble was, much as we loved our house, 'Salud' was now more than we needed, most of the time anyway, with the family away at school and college. Without their help, the big, wild garden was getting even wilder. The house needed central heating and decorating throughout inside as well. We couldn't afford all that yet, we didn't really want to move and the children must have a home to come back to.

This had got to be the answer: cut the garden in half, build a house at the bottom and sell 'Salud' to pay for it. Surely, as we already owned the land, the cost and what we got from the sale would balance out – especially if the boys and Sarah helped with some of the outside work involved, in their holidays. What would Elisabeth say to the idea? Of course, we mightn't get planning permission anyway – the whole thing might founder on a number of rocks – but – it was worth a go! . . .

A smell of burning came through the vents of the car and caught me in the throat. I stared round. A hundred yards off to my left smoke was pouring from the upper windows of a big house. I hadn't spotted it before. I had been too preoccupied with my own thoughts. I slowed down and watched. With a muffled roar, flames burst through every aperture: the roof disintegrated and the fire soared skyward. It had been a huge monstrosity of a house, empty for years and vandalized beyond renovation but still, there was something sad and awe-inspiring about seeing it being gutted before my eyes.

I stopped the car, got out and began walking towards the blaze. Who had set it alight, I wondered? Then I remembered seeing some lorries parked there the day before and now I could see a group of men standing near a car, just out of range of the heat and falling sparks. The roof timbers fell

74

in as I approached. The tallest man in the group seemed to be in charge. 'What happened?' I asked him.

'We're pulling the place down for a building site. Timbers were rotted and worm-eaten. Easiest way to get rid of the structure.'

I had a sudden brainwave. 'Any chance of buying some hard core? I asked the big man.

'Hard core's valuable stuff,' he said. 'How much would you be wanting?'

Hard core's not my usual fare, so to speak, but I tried to look as if buying it was a habit of mine, did a quick mental calculation and said firmly, 'Fifty yards would do.'

He glanced at me with more respect and said, 'Hmm. I could manage that. Where do you want it hauled? That's where the cost comes.'

'Only round the corner and up the farm road.'

'Well, that's a help – let you have it for a pound a yard.'

I knew enough to realize that that was a lot less than the normal price and I guessed that in fact he would be quite glad to be shot of it. 'How soon will you want to know definitely?' I asked.

'Pulling the walls down tomorrow,' he said. 'Give you three days, maximum.'

As I went on up the lane home I was feeling a mixture of elation and apprehension. We would need that hard core for a drive to the new house that hadn't even existed in my mind a quarter of an hour before. Hadn't I jumped the gun? What on earth was Elisabeth going to say? Yet – all that lovely hard core, cheap and handy – I couldn't just ignore it!

It comforted me to remember that we hadn't just been relying on our own ideas, we had been praying about the future. We genuinely wanted to do what we believed God wanted for us. But what about that parable – pulling down barns to build greater? Well, it wasn't our barn that had got pulled down, and we would be building something lesser with cheaper running costs and a lot less work too.

Elisabeth is unpredictable. She didn't say anything in response to my wildcat scheme, not until next morning. I was well into the toast and marmalade when she said, 'OK then.'

'OK what?' I asked.

'OK to the building idea. Let's try it and see what happens.'

The next few weeks were a bit of a blur, made up largely of town planning permits, solicitor's documents, house agents, potential buyers who turned out to be sightseers, and then at last, a genuine purchaser.

But who was going to do the building? And what sort of a house was he going to build? Books of plans and reams of squared paper later, the idea evolved of an L-shaped bungalow built around the pond Peter had designed years before – a sun-trap facing south with the kitchen window facing north so that we could look at the Downs while we washed up.

An architect obligingly took our crude sketches, and under his hand, the drawing of a ranch-house with picture windows, a steep roof and a tall chimney-stack appeared as if by magic. But – still no builder. We didn't want a big, expensive, impersonal firm but a small man who would really take an interest and not too much of a chunk out of ou slender resources.

It was then that Bill Stanton appeared in the surgery one morning. A cheerful, chatty chap was Bill.

'Just lifting a bag of cement off the pile, wasn't I? Then – bingo – just like someone was sticking a knife in me guts, wasn't it? Found this here lump in me groin next morning, didn't I?' He made all his announcements in this sort of rhetorical question form. A lump he had indeed, one which disappeared with steady compression and reappeared when I made him cough.

'Got yourself a nice hernia, haven't you?' I seemed to be catching the same habit. 'Need an operation.'

'Ain't that just me luck? And we're bang in the middle of a job, aren't we? Could have done without this lot, couldn't I?'

'What job are you on?' I asked.

'Buildin' a garage for a bloke, aren't we? Dunno what the

gaffer's goin' to say. Have to get a stand-in, won't he, that's all? How long will it take, doc?'

'About a week in hospital and then about six weeks before you do much lifting.' I let it sink in. 'Do any house building?' I asked casually.

'Lots,' he said. 'Know the manager of the bank in the square? Did one for him last year, didn't we?'

I began a letter to McFarlane, the surgeon; as I finished, I looked up again at Bill Stanton.

'What's your gaffer's name, Bill?'

'Jack Major. Going to do his nut, isn't he? Six blinking weeks on the panel!'

'At least,' I said. I was thinking, 'The house that Jack built,' silly, I know, but it was rather a coincidence.

'We're partners really,' said Bill, interrupting my train of thought. 'Only he's the tradesman and I'm his mate like, aren't I?'

We contacted the bank manager and he very kindly said we were welcome to take a look at his house. He sounded quite proud of it.

'Bit rough here and there, you know, but we're very satisfied, on the whole. Worked like beavers, those two.'

It sounded good enough to us. I arranged to meet Jack and he perused my plans with a critical eye.

'Hm, not bad,' he conceded, with condescension. 'That roof though, that'd fall in for a start. Needs much stronger purlins. Four by twos – huh!' he snorted.

I nodded, wondering what a purlin was.

'Don't mind 'avin' a go. Be wantin' an estimate, won't you? I'll give you that, but no commitments like. We work by the hour, you pay for materials, but I'll see you get trade prices, mind you.'

We were to learn that for all his taciturnity, Jack was always on our side. Woe betide the suppliers who sent anything not up to scratch. 'You can just take that lot straight back,' he would say to the flabbergasted truck-driver, over what seemed to me a perfectly satisfactory load of timber. 'Think they can fool me,' he would say. 'Been too long at the game for that.'

The estimate, large though it seemed to us who had never built with anything more expensive than mud-bricks and local timber from the forests of Kenya, was almost exactly what we hoped we'd cleared for the sale of 'Salud.'

'Start when Bill gets back,' said Jack. "Avin' a 'oliday, 'e is, I reckon 'e done it on purpose.'

That gave us six weeks to get that drive done. Fortunately the family were at home, so we set about the back-breaking task of laying fifty cubic yards of rubble with the aid of a wheelbarrow, a shovel and a rammer or two, the last supplied by our good friend, Buttercup Joe, from his store of junk. That concluded, thirty yards of ready-mixed concrete was delivered in one day and the drive was finished.

As I lay in bed, my biceps bulging like those of a prize fighter and my back feeling as if it had been run over by the tank that Jack, on viewing our handiwork, had sarcastically observed that the drive would now take, I totted up the expense that we had saved. It came to several hundred pounds. We saved some more by buying a stack of handmade bricks at a reduced rate from a patient who ran a country brick-yard, as they were left over from building a church. Jack handled one or two with disdain.

'Just trying to make it difficult for me with this lot, that's what you're doing,' he grumbled. 'All different sizes, see?' But I saw the gleam of a craftsman in his eye at the prospect of handling something with a bit of character in it.

Jack was a large, burley man who wore a cement-impregnated cap perched on a mop of dark, curly hair. In moments of abstraction he would lift his cap and scratch his bald patch with the third finger of the same hand. Bill was spare and wiry. He needed to be. He did a dozen different jobs requiring strength and agility. He mixed the 'pug' – cement and sand – put up scaffolding, painted, carried bricks for Jack and did the accounts, *and* he was the sand-bag to absorb Jack's barbs of wrath when things went wrong. He accomplished it all with an impervious good humour. He mightn't be a tradesman but he earned his half-share, I reckoned.

One thing I never got used to. Suddenly, without warning, just when the work was going nicely, they would quietly disappear for several days. When I groused, Jack would say, 'You get paid whether you've got customers or not, doc. We have to keep ours happy or where would we be when our job 'ere's finished, eh?'

Poor Jack, I tried his patience sorely. 'Just popping down the garden,' I would say to Elisabeth, when I came in for coffee. 'See how they're getting on.'

It became habitual and Jack, seeing me coming, for he had eyes in the back of his head, would strike up his favourite ditty – and he only had one – 'Beautiful Dreamer', and ignore me. Bill, on the other hand, provided he was out of sight round a corner from Jack, was all too willing to lean on his spade (at my expense) and chat.

'Half-way up the ladder, wasn't I. . .

My new vocabulary expanded weekly. 'Pug' I knew, and I rapidly became conversant in footings, headers, courses, raked joints, wall plates, tie-beams, king posts, barge-boards – the lot. A lady who came to the surgery one day with dropped arches gave me a curious look when I inadvertently asked her to remove her shoes so that I could examine her footings.

'You'll 'ave to watch out on your inspections, doc,' said Jack one morning. 'It'll be like a bloomin' battlefield around 'ere when the tilers come – cut your 'ead off if you don't keep your eyes peeled!' He was right. Perched aloft, those young men hurled flawed tiles in any direction with joyous abandon and soon the ground was ankle-deep in shattered tiles. 'Nice bit of 'ard core for the paths,' said Jack.

Very late in the day I had one of my bright ideas. 'Jack,' I said, 'what about tiling the kitchen?' He flung down his trowel, pushed back his cap and said, with unexpected violence, 'See 'ere doc, you can't go putting things in the contract like that right at the last minute. You know, I can pack me tools anytime.' I retreated in confusion. The kitchen was tiled, just the same, without further comment.

When I rose each morning my first thought was to look out of the window at the structure rising up steadily against the background of trees and Downs beyond. Though there were as yet no windows and the woodwork was unpainted, it already presented a comfortable, homely appearance with its pinky-brown church bricks and long low profile.

Concentrating on my real job in life wasn't easy. The practice was busy, but Charles and Fred were very tolerant. Charles even made time to carry out a personal assessment of the progress we were making. Our approach had Jack at full throttle on 'Beautiful Dreamer'. Charles gazed for a minute at our pride and joy and then said drily, 'Yes, I can see building houses is more in your line. Pity you didn't stick to it.'

'There's a call for Miss Peckwharton,' said Mrs Banbury on my return to the surgery. 'Perhaps you could make it your first.'

Mrs Banbury was getting the knack of sorting the urgent from the trivial, and she was absolutely right this time. A neighbour was awaiting me anxiously. 'Don't like the look of her, doctor.'

I didn't either. She was breathing very quickly and her lips had a nasty blue tinge. 'Only really a cold on the chest,' she assured me.

She showed all the signs of bronchitis when I examined her, but there was something else too. There was a nasty rumble and slap in one area of her heart-sounds.

'Did you ever have rheumatic fever as a child?' I asked.

'Yes, as a matter of fact I did. I was in bed for weeks. Afterwards I was told I had a weak heart and mustn't play strenuous games. That's really why I took to writing.' I hadn't realized she was a writer. Anyway, she had valvular damage in her heart and the bronchitis had put extra strain on it. I gave her some tablets for her heart and congestion, and an antibiotic, taking some sputum in a tube for bacterial examination as well. When I had written the prescription for the neighbour to get from the chemist, I turned to Miss Peckwharton again.

'What do you write?'

'There are some of my books on the piano downstairs.' I thought she blushed slightly, but the light was bad in the bedroom. On my way out I had a look on the piano, but I could only find a pile of paperback Westerns by 'Wilbur T. Hardacre'; *Gunfight at Big C Corrall, Kid Carson Rides Again, Rustlers of Red Gulch* and similar uplifting titles. I picked up one or two and nipped back up the stairs. 'These are all I can find.'

'Yes, they're all mine.'

'You write Westerns?' I said, unable to hide my disbelief.

'Yes, before you stands, or lies, I should say, "Wilbur T. Hardacre." It's not so difficult, though I've never been farther west than Llandudno. I subscribe to a magazine of cowboy history and folk lore, and I look up information about firearms in the public library. They sell very well, my books', she added, 'even in Arizona! It's a welcome addition to my pension, the royalties, and . . .' here she hesitated, 'I'm able to help my cousin who's a missionary nurse in Thailand.'

'Now I've heard everything,' I thought as I went down the stairs. Here was a lady of sixty-seven writing Westerns to help her cousin do missionary work – that really beat the lot.

I got back in time after afternoon surgery to take the men's tray down the garden. Jack and Bill seated themselves on boxes which had housed the kitchen sink unit and drank their tea. I'd brought a mug for myself.

Ever read anything by Wilbur T. Hardacre?' I asked casually.

Bill looked at me. 'I've not long finished *The Lone Rider of Deadman's Canyon*. Why, doc?'

'Oh, just that I've met the author.'

'Go on – you never! What's he like then? Sunburned and all diamond rings?'

'No, just ordinary like you and me. Not a bit like you would expect – but clever, very clever.' I wasn't going to blow Miss Peckwharton's cover and maybe cause a fall in her sales. I was quite glad when Jack started asking me about what sort of taps we wanted.

As I took my routine early-morning survey through the bedroom window I said thoughtfully to Elisabeth, still under the bedclothes, 'What are we going to call it then, the new house?'

Names mean a lot to Elisabeth, perhaps they do to me too. Particularly houses and people. No dice though, that morning, we couldn't think of a suitable title for our new home. The week went by – surgeries, visits, house inspections and on Friday I was due to see Johnny Taggerty again. He was much better, quite cheeky and wanting a dose of nursery rhymes plus pin-men.

'Tell me the cow with the cwumpled horn wiv pitchers,' he insisted. Obediently I repeated the whole thing; 'the farmer, the cock, the priest, the man, the maiden, the cow,' right through to the end, then he wanted it all over again. I'd got as far as 'the cock that crowed in the morn' when the penny dropped. 'Cockcrow'! Why not call the house 'Cockcrow'? There was 'Cockcrow Bottom', a wooded valley in the Downs; Jesus' disciple, Peter, was warned of his denial of his Master by the cock crowing and Jesus himself had said we must be ready for his return at any time – it might be at cock-crow. A name like that would keep us on our toes. Elisabeth liked it too.

'Wot yer goin' to call this 'ere domicile of yours, doc?' Jack was all smiles. The last brick had been laid on the chimney and he was due for a hand-out to celebrate 'topping-out'.

'Cockcrow.'

'Cockcrow? Wot d'you want to call it that for?'

'Well, that's when doctors often have to get up.'

'Go on! Bet I'm up before you most days, doc.'

'A cock crowed when Peter the disciple said he didn't know Jesus. It'll help us not to forget that.'

Jack pushed his cap back and scratched the bald patch. 'Takes all sorts, doc,' he said at last.

I had been on duty all weekend so I had Monday afternoon off. Jack let me hold the other end of boards for him and I was really enjoying myself when Elisabeth came down the garden.

'Sorry, love,' she whispered, 'A couple, foster-parents, from down the lane, have brought a little boy . . .' She only

,ot as far as that when a procession hove in sight down the ﹒iew drive. 'I did *ask* them to wait,' said Elisabeth.

The lady was in the lead. Behind her came the man and the boy. The man was carrying a bottle and as they got close I could see that the boy kept near the bottle – very near in fact, as his tongue was stuck in the neck. It was a situation you meet infrequently – possibly about once in a hundred years.

'He was sticking his tongue down while he was sucking the lemonade,' said the lady, and there was indeed residue of nasty-looking yellow liquid in the bottom of the bottle, 'then he couldn't get his tongue out.'

I examined his tongue. It was constricted in the narrow part of the neck and then swollen and oedematous-looking where the neck widened out. Fortunately, and I said an inward 'thank you' for it, it was a plastic bottle; a glass one would have presented horrific possibilities in any attempt to remove it.

I was debating a course of action when Jack volunteered, 'Got an idea, doc.' He and Bill had quietly joined the party. He walked very deliberately back into the new house and emerged with something in his hand.

'Now, son,' his voice was very gentle, 'let this old gaffer have a look at you.' The little fellow looked up with eyes that were red from crying and he seemed to respond trustfully to Jack.

'Come and sit down 'ere,' Jack went on. He got the boy sitting on the garden-seat, with his head on Jack's knee and Jack's foot up on the seat. Then he revealed a little hacksaw, sawed off the bottom of the bottle, and from his overall pocket he took a pair of tin snips and dextrously chopped through the bottle all the way up to the rim of the neck, carefully avoiding catching the lad's tongue in the process. Last of all he seized the two sides in his powerful hands, prized the bottle open and, hey presto, out came the boy's tongue. Elisabeth took him into the kitchen and he was soon happily drinking iced milk with his tongue rapidly resuming its normal size and shape.

I went out again to the back of the new house, whence

'Beautiful Dreamer' was gently carrying on the breeze towards me.

'Thanks, Jack, you were great.'

'Any time, doc. Always fancied me chances as a surgeon.'

Perhaps it was one little boy that made me think of the other, perhaps it was Jack's kindness. Whatever it was, I went and fetched Johnny Taggerty the next day to show him 'the house that Jack built.' As we drove the car up the drive, I stopped and pointed to the weathercock I'd persuaded Jack to fix to the gable-end.

'Look, Johnny, the cock that crowed in the morn.' He lifted his eyes with their unhealthy, blue-pouched lower lids and stared up through the windscreen.

'He dun't crow, doctor, does he?'

'No, Johnny, he's only a 'tending cock.'

I lifted Johnny's flimsy weight from the car into the hallway where Jack was nailing down floorboards. 'This is Jack, who built the house.'

''Ullo, mate,' said Jack, and stuck out a massive hand to take the boy's frail white one. After that I took him out quickly. Bill had come to greet him too, and I was afraid Johnny might think he was 'the man, all tattered and torn', for he did have an enormous rent in the seat of his overalls.

Johnny had final thrill on the way home. We had to wait at the bottom of the drive for a herd of Farmer Jenkins's milking cows to pass and there at the end was a cow with one twisted horn, which had somehow escaped cauterization in calfhood, hanging down almost over one eye. Johnny spotted it.

'Cow with cwumpled horn, doctor, look, cow with cwumpled horn.'

The day finally came when Jack did pack his tools and Bill scraped pug off his shovel for the last time and cleaned his paintbrushes.

Jack stood back and looked at his creation.

'Thank goodness that job's finished. No more 'omemade bricks or funny tiles. Shan't be comin' back 'ere no more, doc, I can tell you. I've 'ad enough of workin' in the backwoods.'

Two weeks later, there was a toot of a horn on the drive. It was Jack. 'This is my missus, doc. Thought I ought to show 'er the awful place you made me build.'

He showed her round with ill-concealed pride and they stayed for tea in the lounge, looking out at Peter's pond, twinkling and shining in the afternoon sun. As they drove off down the drive, Elisabeth and I stood in the doorway. I put my arm round her waist.

'Look at "Salud", I said. 'It doesn't seem to mind.' Its brown roof looked comfortably at us over the fence and from our old garden came the shouts of children.

10

Angel on a moped

'Is that Doctor Hamilton? Sorry to ring you at home at this hour, doctor. This is Nurse Marden. I'm worried about an old lady I'm looking after. She is one of your patients. I would be grateful for your advice. I could meet you here if you could manage it?'

It was only a quarter to nine in the morning and it was an unusual way of doing things – but then I'd already realized on the occasions when I'd met her that there wasn't much that was usual about Nurse Marden. The normal procedure would have been for me to be called to see the patient and then to have asked for nursing help if required.

'Right. As it happens, I *am* on visits today. I'll come at once. Where are you?'

'Fine, doctor. I'm at 47 Parklands. It's Mrs Fairbairn. I'll be waiting for you – see you.'

The vicar of our church, Algernon Greenfield, had warned me about Mary.

'Doctor, she's a one-off. You'll never meet another like her.' That was good coming from Algernon, who was the original eccentric himself. I suppose he could recognize a rival at forty paces. He went on jovially, 'the normal isn't to be expected from Mary Marden.'

Nurse Marden was in her fifties, having 'retired' to Wilverton after a long period of service as a missionary nurse in Tel Aviv. She had seen the creation of the Jewish State of Israel, and witnessed the grim activities of Irgun Zwi Leumi and the Stern gang. She ministered impartially to Arab and Jew alike amid great danger, with, I imagine, a cool head and a lot of good humour. Now in 'retirement', she was tearing round the hills – and there are seven of them in Wilverton, like Rome – on an ancient moped, doing nursing for needy folk for next to nothing.

Elisabeth and I had first met her one Sunday morning after church. We were struck by her big blue eyes, sparkling with mischief, her charming face and a mop of unruly grey curls. As we drove home, Elisabeth had said to me, 'Why on earth didn't some undeserving male snap her up years ago?'

'Beats me. Lucky I met you first!'

Elisabeth had laughed. 'You were hardly out of short trousers when she was around!'

'Doctor,' said Mary, now dressed in a smart blue uniform and felt hat as she opened the big front door of the Victorian house to me, 'it's not Mrs Fairbairn I am really worried about. She's a widow needing a leg ulcer treated. She got my name somehow and had a neighbour call me as she wanted private nursing and didn't want to bother you. She's getting on fine, ulcer's healing nicely. But would you have a look, as she's your patient? No, it's her brother I'm worried about, but I've never seen him.'

I thought that was a bit cryptic.

'If you've never seen him, what are you worried about?' I asked, genuinely puzzled.

'Well, he's here upstairs – permanently – never comes down. You hear him moving about – that is, we did until today and that worries me even more. But there is a most terrible pong drifting downwards – worse than the back streets of Jerusalem on a warm day. I thought you ought to know. He's a patient of yours too.'

She was right not to mince words about the 'pong': a sort of miasma, reminiscent of rotting cabbages, laced with burning paraffin and a touch of very elderly damp socks wound its way round the lower reaches of the staircase from the gloom above. Mrs Fairbairn herself had made a bedroom out of the big downstairs dining-room as she couldn't go upstairs any more.

I introduced myself and examined her leg. Right enough, she had a large varicose ulcer but under Mary's treatment it was healed half-way across.

'Getting good treatment, I see, Mrs Fairbairn. Carry on –
you're doing fine.'

'Doctor, has Nurse Marden told you about Laurence, my
brother? He is, I think the word is, a "recluse". His landlord
threw him out from his flat in Wimbledon so I took him in.
Tradesmen deliver his food upstairs and I never see him. We
are worried in case he's not well or something. Would you
be good enough to give him a call? I can't get up the stairs
now myself and I didn't like to ask Nurse Marden.'

'Certainly, I'll go up now.'

The smell got stronger as I went up the stairs followed by
Mary. There was a dull beam of light under one of the front
room doors. I knocked. There was no reply, so I opened the
door and a wall of stale, stinking air hit us in the face.

I've been in some scenes of filth and disorder but never
one like this.

A naked bulb shone dimly in the misty atmosphere.
Opened tins, half-empty, lay scattered over the floor; blackened cooking pots with mildewed contents lay in the
fireplace; filthy bedding lay heaped on the bed and over
everything lay a pall of dust; an oil stove, ill-adjusted, sent
out smokey black fumes into the air – but there was no one
to be seen!

Suddenly, as from a void, a voice spoke – a curiously high-
pitched but educated and rather stilted voice:

'To whom do I owe the honour of this unsolicited but
nonetheless welcome visitation to my humble abode?'

Mary was beside me and our eyes scanned the room.
Amid the chaos I suddenly spotted two scrawny bare legs
protruding slightly from under the bed, the rest of the body
being concealed by an old eiderdown hanging drukenly over
the edge. I stepped cautiously but quickly across the floor
and knelt to peer under the bed.

There was an old man of about seventy-five, naked from
the waist down with a greyish-coloured vest covering his
upper half, lying, quite calmly, with his head on a pair of
dilapidated carpet slippers. The state of the floor around him
was indescribable.

'I'm Doctor Hamilton. What are you doing under there?'

'Good morning to you, doctor. May I offer you my apologies for a lamentable lack of the normal courtesies to be extended to one's medical adviser on his attendance. May I assure you that my adoption of this present unusual posture is of a quite involuntary nature. To be precise, I slipped while performing my ablutions and descended hither and find myself unable to regain sufficient equilibrium to extract myself.'

'Nurse,' I said over my shoulder, 'lend me a hand.'

Half-naked old men don't alarm Nurse Marden; she seized the poor fellow and together we manoeuvred him on to a blanket and then dragged him out from under the bed, without getting splinters in his hindquarters.

He was very cold. But for the burning oil stove, he would have been dead from hypothermia and exhaustion. I could find no evidence that he had hit his head or been unconscious, but he was suffering badly from exposure and lack of food and water. We lifted him onto the bed and I left Mary attending to him as best she could amidst all the rubbish of the room, while I went down to Mrs Fairbairn.

'We found that your brother had had a fall and we're looking after him, but I think he ought to go into a nursing home at once. Has he the means to pay the charges?'

'Don't worry about that, doctor. He only has the old age pension and assistance, but I can manage any bills. Won't you use my phone?' She had one by the bed.

I knew that Langport Nursing Home was efficient and kind. They had a single room available, thank goodness. I didn't imagine anyone would put up with the flow of archiac conversation for long in a shared room. I gave them the rundown on his condition. 'And I'll call to see Mr Grantham tomorrow,' I finished.

Mary had already got him cleaned up and warm in his bed. I had heard her coming down to get a hot-water bottle filled in the kitchen while I was phoning.

When I called at the Langport in the afternoon next day I beheld a transformation. Seated in an old-fashioned, high-backed, winged armchair sat a distinguished-looking spare old gentleman. He was quietly smoking a long-stemmed briar pipe and wearing a faded but well-made, old-style smoking jacket with gold facings. On his head was a dark red fez with a tassel hanging down over one of his ears.

He bowed graciously to me. After a very formal greeting he continued.

'My dear doctor, I feel I cannot let this occasion pass without an adequate expression of the gratefulness and warmth I feel for the opportune and magnanimous assistance which you and the young lady' (that should please Mary Marden, I thought) 'extended to me in my hour of need. Were it within my power to tender a more concrete expression of my appreciation to you both, I would so do; sadly circumstances do not permit it.' He paused to gather breath.

'That's fine, Mr Grantham, don't give it a thought,' I chipped in. My visiting time was slipping by. 'Any time you're under a bed and need help, don't hesitate to get in touch – but make sure you take a telephone with you!'

The old gentleman, who obviously lived in his mind in another century and had the courtesies of it engraved there, lived on happily in the nursing home to the end of his days. He was an avid reader of the Bible, preferring the *Authorized Version*. Dickens was his other love, and he was like a Dickens character himself.

Nurse Marden chuckled when I told her how he was. 'I've seen some in my time,' she said, 'but never one like him!'

I got on with Mary Marden like a house on fire, but I wondered if our friendship was being stretched a bit when she rang me again – this time mid-morning when I was in the middle of surgery.

'Doc, I'm sorry to be a pest, but there's trouble. Remember Mrs Fairbairn? Well, this isn't medical, it may well be a police job, but I thought I'd get in touch with you. There's a jobbing gardener who's been doing some work for her, and I think he's a crook. Can you help?'

This was an odd sort of request, but Mary Marden is an odd sort of person, as I'd found out.

I went round to Mrs Fairbairn's that afternoon and it was just as well I did. Mary was in an extraordinary condition;

her uniform was torn, her hair all over the place and she had a huge, ugly bruise on the side of her face.

'What on earth's happened?' I said.

She sat down in a chair in the hall and laughed – there was a touch of hysteria in it.

'Doctor, we've had a right party! It's Anderson, the gardener. I suspected him of stealing from Mrs Fairbairn, as I said. He is only a jobbing type and he's done practically nothing that I can see in the garden. Well, I left my bike down the road this afternoon, out of sight behind a hedge, and came back to lie in wait until you came in the little dressing-room that opens off the bedroom, just in case he came back. I knew you were coming so I wasn't too worried.

'Well, sure enough, he came sneaking in, to speak to Mrs Fairbairn. I had the door ajar. When I peeped through, I could see him rifling her purse on the sideboard, while she was looking out of the window. He'd asked her to inspect what he'd done – for the first time, he'd really done some work in the front garden.

'I nipped in and confronted him but he made a break for it. I tried to stop him but he tore my dress and hit me here.' She touched the bruise gingerly. 'He's gone, but he's left his bike in the shed round the side. He must have panicked and just run off, so I locked the shed and here's the key.

I couldn't speak for a moment. Then I said, 'Mary, you are crazy. You should have just let him go.'

Tough as she was, the incident with Anderson had taken it out of Mary and she began to cry quietly. I asked Mrs Fairbairn if I could make some tea. She seemed only partly aware of what had happened.

While the kettle was boiling, I rang the police. I got my old friend Inspector Dai Jones, and related the events of the morning to him. The Wilverton police traced the bicycle, caught Fred Anderson (which wasn't his real name) and he received a term in gaol for his exploits. It turned out that he had a record of several previous convictions for burglary, assault and grievous bodily harm. But he'd obviously met his match in the 'angel on a moped!'

11
Marram grass

'Doctor Hamilton, how much would it cost to fit the ward with proper bed curtains?' He was deliberately keeping his voice low. I looked at the emaciated man in the bed and wondered what was in his mind.

'I really couldn't say – oh, Sister, could you spare a minute?'

The pleasant-faced ward sister halted in her rapid progress down the ward.

'What can I do for you, doctor?'

'Mr Rigby here has a question for you, sister.'

She looked enquiringly at Frank Rigby. With an effort he shifted himself up the bed and said again in a conspiratorial whisper, 'What would it cost to fit this ward with proper curtains for each bed?'

Sister glanced around, taking in the sixteen beds and the unwieldy screens on castors round several beds where intimate procedures were taking place.

'We-e-ll, I should guess . . . properly done . . . about fifty pounds a bed – that's including material, the making, all the fittings and the like. Yes, probably fifty pounds a bed.'

Rigby was quietly working it out. 'Eight hundred pounds then, or say a thousand – just to allow for extras. Hmmm.'

'What are you on about, Mr Rigby?' asked sister.

'Oh, nothing much,' was all he would say.

I'd nearly finished my hospital round of visits to patients. I wasn't able to get in very often but Rigby was a bit special. I'd been seeing a lot of him over the past few months.

He was a strange, awkward chap and he had a slight stutter. He was unmarried and had lived with his elderly mother until six months previously when suddenly she had died. As a chief mechanic on RAF bombers he had had a nice secure job but had taken an early discharge to come home to look after his elderly mother. He had registered with the practice on coming home but had never been to the surgery. With his expertise in electronics, he had soon picked up a job as a top technician in the telephone service.

After his mother's death he decided he had to do something about the cough he had which just wouldn't clear up. We had him X-rayed, and a tell-tale shadow had shown up on one lung. Admission to a London chest hospital followed, and there he had a partial pneumonectomy – removal of part of the lung. He had had carcinoma of a bronchus – cancer of an air-passage of the lung.

He had made a good recovery and had gone to convalesce in his beloved Norfolk, spending his time peacefully motorboating on the Broads, which in those days hadn't become a new sort of traffic hazard area. His father had owned a yacht and cruiser-hiring business but he had died while Rigby was quite young. His mother had sold up and come to live in Wilverton as it was warmer for her than the breezy east coast, but Frank had never lost his love of those sweeps of fenland and the great expanses of open water.

When we had first met we had had a good laugh together. It was one of those occasions when you discover an amazing crossing of paths.

'Which yacht did your father let out?' I asked one day when he had told me where he'd come from.

'The *Goldens*,' he said. '*Golden Plover*, *Golden Hind*, *Golden Eagle* – those were some of them.'

I sat back and laughed. 'You won't believe this, Frank, but I sailed in the *Golden Hind* with a crew of boys before the war. I say "sailed" – I sailed it right back into your dad's boat-shed with masts and sails up. Thought I could come back into the cut with a following wind because it was almost a dead calm. I hadn't reckoned it would gust round a gap in the trees. It was too late to turn in the cut and the boys jumped ashore with the bow and stern rond anchors to try and hold her up. Couldn't do it in time. The forestay met the shed roof and bounced us backwards, but the jib-sail caught on a nail and tore. You should have heard your dad's language. It wasn't fit for our young ears – but I deserved it. Regular novice's caper, that was.'

He looked at me with a new light in his eyes. At last he spoke. 'I c-can har-hardly believe it. My dad was talking about that to his dying day. Called you all sorts of things he did. He'd only just re-rigged that boat and it was his pride and joy.'

Frank came back looking really fit from his holiday and he went back to his electronics job. Sadly, his recovery wasn't long maintained. One day, just when I thought he would be rebuilding his life and getting used to fending for himself, he came back to see me.

'Not been so good doc – weighed myself this morning. I've lost five pounds!'

This *was* bad news; at the best of times he was a spare individual. Just now, stripped, he looked positively cadaverous.

When I examined him I found some nasty suspicious enlargements of his neck glands. A check with the London hospital revealed a re-occurrence of the whole condition, and further operative or X-ray treatment was out of the question. He was admitted to the Duke of Gloucester for care, and I think I knew that his time was getting short.

Three weeks later he began to go downhill very quickly and then, quite suddenly, he died. A few days before, he had told me wistfully how, as a boy, he sometimes used to cycle on Sundays to a little Methodist chapel near the village of Horsey on the Broads. He told me about the sermons he listened to from local farmers and others. One man he liked especially was a simple chap whose work was making baskets from the osiers cut from pollarded willows along the roads and dykes in that part of the world.

'I remember him saying that faith in Jesus was like the framework of a basket and our living was what you wove out of the framework. I've still got the framework,' he added, 'but the rest of the basket has got rather neglected.'

Maybe it's true that 'the evil that men do lives after them, the good is oft interred with their bones', but that didn't happen in Frank Rigby's case. . .

Elisabeth and I sat at breakfast looking at a letter that had come in the morning's mail. It was the bill for Peter's term at boarding school: £150.

'We haven't that in the kitty,' I said. 'Not until next month's pay-day. We aren't going to be able to go away on a holiday this year either, I'm afraid.'

I looked at the rest of the post. There was a long, good quality envelope which I opened next.

'Well, what do you know! Look at this.'

It was from a firm of solicitors: 'We are pleased to inform you that in the Will of Frank Rigby Esq deceased he has left you the sum of Two Hundred Pounds.'

Tears came to my eyes. 'Fancy old Frank thinking of us.'

That these two letters came in the same post was remarkable, but what made it quite extraordinary was the third – from Elisabeth's sister, Christine: 'I am trying to get a family party together to rent a farm on the edge of the Broads in September. We could hire four or five half-deckers and moor them on the nearby cut. Do come – it would be very cheap, and lovely to get together.'

'Can we manage it, Andy?' said Elisabeth. I'd love the children to meet their cousins and I know they'd like sailing.'

'We can now,' I said. 'There'll still be some over from Frank Rigby's legacy.'

We felt very proud to be singled out for remembrance by Frank but we were taken down a peg or two when the local paper came through the door. Frank's bequests had made quite a story. It was headed, 'Lone ex-RAF man remembers his many friends.' There followed an amazing list of legacies that he had made, headed by £1,000 to the D.O.G.S. to provide curtains for D Ward. He had remembered both my partners as he had me. The lady who cleaned for him, some of his mates at work, his postman, even the man who came to lay the carpet for him in his home – none had been forgotten.

It was curiously fitting that Frank's kindness should enable us to go to the Broads that he loved, when he couldn't go himself any more.

The evenings were getting a little shorter when we drove off to Norfolk. We towed our caravan all the way. At last, in the late afternoon, we turned off a little broad-land road, lined with dykes and willows, on to a path running across rough pasture towards a thatched building lying snugly beneath the dunes on a coast near Horsey. Standing on the track, waving, was Christine.

We were the first to arrive but, by nightfall, family party after family party had come and been given their berths in the old farmhouse or the converted stables or they had fixed themselves up in tents or caravans. We had all brought sleeping bags and Christine had ordered and collected a mass of food from the village shop.

With thirty of us to cater for, it was an absolute essential to fix a rota for washing-up, cooking, fetching milk and provisions, for getting water from the pump outside the kitchen door, for emptying the chemical loo and for sundry clearing-up jobs round the place.

As the farmhouse was virtually standing at the foot of sand dunes while beyond lay the sea, the well water that we pumped had an interesting selection of flavours, ranging from a touch of swamp water to good old briny. We boiled every drop before we used it. After a few days we began to notice that a new flavour had crept in. A minty one. This remained a mystery until one morning I happened to spot the oldest member of the party emptying her tooth-mug into the grating beneath the pump-spout.

'I say, that goes straight back into the well, you know!' I exclaimed.

'Oh, my dear, I thought it was a drain!'

To save labour and money we settled for a cheap and simple diet: largely wholemeal bread with cheese, milk and fruit from a nearby farm at lunch-time, with sausages or bacon and eggs and vegetables for evening meals. We did have the occasional 'bonus': our elevenses were enhanced by the find of an unbroken one-pound tin of Nescafé washed up on the beach. And on a very low tide, we went shrimping and our reward was a bucket full of shrimps for tea.

There was a wonderful selection of wildlife. Peter spent a large amount of time watching the ducks and other water-birds, but the highlight of the holiday for him was the finding by the early morning bathers of a baby seal, with huge, melting black eyes, lying stranded on the beach. He looked at us with faint interest. We left him to be sought out and guided back to the water by his mother, who was bobbing about fifty yards out in the surf.

Every morning a conference was held with plans A, B, C, D and E considered for the day's operations. We had those half-deckers moored on a cut leading on to Horsey Mere, and the whole 200-mile complex of sailing water lay before us.

'I think we should try and get to Barton today,' said Uncle John.

'What about a trip to Yarmouth?' said Uncle Bill.

'I suggest having a shot at the regatta at Potter Heigham,' said cousin David.

'And I suggest a day on the beach,' said Auntie Liz, who was not over-enamoured of sitting on slatted seats for several hours in an unstable small boat.

In the end, as it was getting late, we settled for a look in at the regatta and, if that turned out to be not to our liking, we would try to get on to Yarmouth. Of course, if we had had one skipper instead of eight we might have got off before ten-thirty – but the sandwiches had to be made and the breakfast washed up anyway.

We arrived at the regatta at the last minute and our entry was accepted. Most of the contestants had beautiful, sleek racing dinghies, and our threat to their supremacy in our heavy, old clinker-built fourteen-footer was not very great. We got just clear the edge of the line of bungalows at Potter Heigham Reach when we were met by the leading boats on their return journey to the starting-line. Rather than face the embarrassment of arriving about an hour after the leaders, we continued on our way towards Yarmouth.

It was a blissful fortnight, taken up with sailing, talking

97

and wandering along the wide expanse of shore-line. Each evening we had an impromptu sing-song with all the old sea shanties and folk songs. We would end with a chorus, such as 'This little light of mine', and family prayers. Other old friends of the family had somehow scented us out and were camped nearby. One of them was Tony who was the vicar in charge of the church in Leeds, famous for the hospitality of its crypt to 'gentlemen of the road', such as my hospital companion, Arnold Gadsby.

On Saturday night, we went far and wide collecting firewood and anyone interested, who was camped nearby, for a camp-fire, sing-song and sausage barbecue to be held on the dunes after dark. About sixty turned up. In the fading light of a September evening, we spent a full two hours singing, reciting family 'party pieces' and eating.

At the end Tony, the parson, stood up, ankle-deep in the sand, and told us a parable of the marram grass, which grew all round us on the dunes.

'It's not much of a plant to look at, is it, but it does a vital job. It spreads and sends its roots deep down to find the moisture and so it holds the shifting sands together against the inroads of the sea, which could otherwise break through and drown the fields beyond.

'The world's like the shifting sand,' he said, 'uncertain and unstable and easily overcome by tides of evil and conflict. Each Christian and each Christian home is like a tuft of marram grass, existing in a hostile environment, helping to hold together society's shifting sand, while sending their roots deep to the living water of Jesus Christ. Let's be sure that we have our roots in Christ.' He said a prayer for us all.

The fire had died down, but its embers still glowed. It was quite dark over the dunes; the sea swished and rasped on the beach below. Quietly, folk got to their feet, hand torches were switched on and a thoughtful trek began, back to the scattered little lights of caravans, buildings and tents along the landward side of the sandy slopes.

On Sunday the little local Methodist chapel, anticipating the influx of visitors had thoughtfully put a large tarpaulin over scaffolding at the side of the tiny building so that, with

98

the windows open, the double-sized congregation could all take part in the service. The regular members graciously occupied the seats under the tarpaulin and allowed the visitors the use of the chapel itself, but there was one man who remained seated in the pew at the back – an ancient man with apple cheeks. We discovered he was the king of the Basketmakers', now retired, whom Frank Rigby had known in his boyhood days.

At the end of the second week we had a grand calculation of all expenditure and worked out the cost per head. It was unbelievably small for our family. For two weeks, with our share of the rent of the old farm, the cost of food and the hire of boats, we had just fifty pounds to pay – exactly the amount we had left over from Frank Rigby's legacy after Peter's school fees had been paid.

'Wasn't it kind of Mr Rigby to think of us when he died?' said Sarah, as we drove through the Essex countryside.

'Yes. And wouldn't he be glad to know that he gave us such a happy time together in his own home-county?' said Elisabeth.

12

Broken branch

We all make mistakes, and I admit that my brilliant idea of establishing a branch surgery in an outlying village was one of them. Yet, at the time, it seemed a winner – a really good scheme.

Mrs Higginbotham, a widow, didn't really need all the rooms in her cottage now her family were gone. So I asked her what she thought about the idea of being invaded for two hours every afternoon. There would be a small consideration to augment her pension. She hesitated at first, but then she said, 'They're all folk from the village that I know anyway, doctor. Yes, I could do it.'

If she hadn't been a lady who knew how to keep her mouth shut, I wouldn't have suggested it, but she realized that when, for instance, Mrs Furze came in for treatment to a black eye – because her old man had come home from *The Fox and Hounds* as usual in a belligerent mood – this was something you didn't talk to the neighbours about. You left it to them to do their own dirty work.

We didn't have an auspicious start for our first surgery. As Mrs Furze came in, I gave her what I innocently thought was my normal smile of welcome but it had quite an unexpected effect.

'That's right, doctor, laugh at me. I came here expecting some help and sympathy and mockery's all I get. Well, there's plenty of other doctors about. Good afternoon.'

I understood her feelings – it was a case of kicking the dog. When things go wrong and there's no one else around, you kick the dog. In this instance, I was the only dog handy.

There were repercussions.

'What have you been saying to our Mrs Furze?' asked Charles, waving a National Health card accusingly in my face. She's took herself off our list.' When Charles misuses his native tongue I know he is a mite put out.

'Charles,' I said. 'You just can't win. I only smiled at her in a friendly way.'

'Well, if you smiled like that,' said Charles, 'I can understand it.'

So perhaps our taking Mrs Higginbotham's parlour and sitting-room for reception and interview-room wasn't going to be such a success, but this was only the beginning, after all.

There were other difficulties. One was that I had to be receptionist as well as doctor, and managing the business side of the practice – such as finding records – is really not my greatest gift. Patients had to wait longer at the Winterham (pronounced 'Winterem') Village Surgery than they did at St Arkel's in Wilverton, which, up until then, had been our only surgery.

But still, it made a nice little set-up. A cosy front room accommodated about ten on cane-bottomed chairs, though only nine were available to the public, as Mrs Higginbotham's cat, Ferdie, always sat on the tenth. Through a little passage lay the sitting-room with the sofa and chairs pushed back, a desk in the window and another door leading to the kitchen where I could wash my hands. It really was very convenient. Patients could be examined on the sofa if I let the end down. There was a good light from the back window which looked on to a tiny little garden with hollyhocks and lavender bushes.

Once the villagers got to know about it they simply flocked in, especially hard-working mothers with their children, and pensioners who could ill afford the local bus company's fare into Wilverton.

To tell the truth, I enjoyed it. I felt like a little king in my own domain. We started at two o'clock and officially I closed the door at three, but with a room-full I seldom finished before four.

I was rather concerned that there was no place to park my car except on the main road of the village. Surgery had barely begun one day and I had just written a prescription for

101

penicillin for the village shoemaker who had pricked his finger with his awl – causing red, tell-tale lines of lympangitis to run up his arm, when the door burst open.

I was annoyed, 'Just a moment, please. I've a patient here. . . .'

I stopped. A dishevelled man in a boiler suit with his cap on his head was pushed into the room by several ladies. Among them I recognized Mrs Clout, Elisabeth's home help, who lived in Winterham. It was she who spoke up.

'Sorry Doctor Hamilton, sorry, but we had to come in. See this man,' she indicated the man in front, who was straightening his cap. 'He was delivering in his van to the greengrocer's just up the road and he knocked his back mudguard into your car. We all saw him and when he looked as if he was going to take off and say nothing about it, we brought him in.'

'Course I wasn't going to sheer off wiv'out tellin' yer, guv. They got it all wrong. OK, so I 'it your car. I'm sorry. 'Ere's me name, Alfred Noggins, and I works for Simpsons, the 'olesale fruit and veg at Guildford, and 'ere's me truck number. Nah – can I get on wiv me job? I'm an hour late for deliverin' along the coast already.'

I went out and inspected my car. The front offside wing was dented. I returned inside where Noggins was still held hostage. After I had given him my name and insurance number on a bit of surgery paper, the loyal villagers, all patients of mine, reluctantly parted to let him through. He departed, grumbling.

'Thank you very much,' I smiled at them.

'That's all right, doctor, sorry for pushing in.' They filed out, headed by Mrs Clout, looking like one who had just seen justice done, but only just.

I had a job to get the firm to settle up. They seemed to think that I was partly to blame for having the effrontery to have my car stationary on the road, but they paid up in the end, without, I imagine, notifying their insurers.

Despite this show of loyalty on the part of the locals and the appreciation they expressed for the local surgery, I found that often they would go either to St Arkel anyway *or* the branch surgery, whichever they felt like. Medical records began to get in a fearful tangle, with half the notes in Winterham and half in Wilverton. After the novelty of having their own surgery began to wear off, numbers attending started to drop. They probably missed combining shopping in Wilverton with getting their 'shopping list' of medicines from the doctor as well.

The other major snag was having no telephone in Mrs Higginbotham's cottage. The village greengrocer just up the road obligingly took emergency calls, but it wasn't the same as my being able to talk direct to Mrs Banbury at the St Arkel surgery.

I was just closing up one Friday afternoon when the green-grocer burst in unceremoniously. His face was red with running and the light in his eyes suggested that he was enjoying being involved in a little drama.

'Doctor,' he gasped. 'You're wanted – urgent. Mr Twistle-ton, 12 Church Lane. Your secretary said to go at once. Heart attack, she said.'

'Thanks.' I grabbed my bag and ran to the car.

It was only a minute or two through the village. The front door of 12 Church Lane was open. In the back room I found Mrs Twistleton holding up her husband in a chair. He was lolling back, his eyes open and his tongue hanging out. He wasn't breathing. I looked at his eyes, the pupils were large and the eyes diverging. I tore open his shirt and listened to his chest. There was no heartbeat.

'Please stand aside,' I said to Mrs Twistleton.

I put my left hand on his chest over his heart and hit it very hard with the butt end of my clenched fist. It could have broken his ribs. It certainly hurt my hand, but he was a heavily-built man of forty-five and I doubted it – anyway, it didn't matter. I listened again. There was a confused throbbing which quickly became a steady impulse. He wasn't going to need cardiac massage. He made a gurgling sound in his throat and then took a strangled gasp. I looked at his eyes – they were converging again and his pupils were getting back to normal size.

I dragged him off the chair, lowered him to the floor and

commenced artificial respiration. Soon he was beginning to draw in the life-giving air himself so that mouth-to-mouth breathing wasn't necessary.

'Get an ambulance – 999. Say "cardiac" – "car-di-ac". I repeated it. I glanced over my shoulder at Mrs Twistleton to make sure she understood. There were tears in her eyes, but she said nothing and slipped out into the hall.

With amazing speed the ambulance men arrived, carrying forced respiration oxygen apparatus. They strapped the mask on Mr Twistleton's face and turned on the oxygen. They waited a moment, then lifted him on to the stretcher and carried him, now semi-conscious, out to the ambulance.

I knew his history; he was an asthmatic, and I began wondering if he had been using his inhaler too frequently. I turned to Mrs Twistleton and asked her.

'Yes, doctor, he had been wheezy and he'd used it a lot more than you told him to. He was just standing hanging a picture when he said he felt queer and collapsed. That's when I called the surgery.'

I wrote down a short history on a piece of paper for the house physician and went out and handed it to the ambulance men. The ambulance roared off. Then I went back into the house. Mrs Twistleton stood there and looked at me.

'Oh, thank you doctor, thank you, thank you.' She looked as if for two pins she would have kissed me.

'Glad I was just round the corner, Mrs Twistleton. He's not out of the woods yet, I'm afraid. But he's alive and that's something.'

As I drove away I found myself in two minds. No telephone at the Winterham surgery was a risk, but if I'd not been in the village at all, Twistleton would have been dead by now. With cardiac arrest, a few more minutes would have been fatal. If I'd had to drive out from Wilverton. . . .

Charles, Fred and I decided that we'd keep it for a year – give it a go and then decide what to do. I'm glad we did, otherwise I would never have met Kirby Langford.

He lived in the village of Winterham about 100 yards from the surgery. He had recently come to retire in the village although he was only fifty-two because he was suffering from the effects of pulmonary tuberculosis which he'd had in his youth. His lungs were now so scarred up that a walk of more than 100 yards would leave him gasping and he would have to sit on a wall and rest. He had never attended the main surgery in Wilverton. A local surgery suited him down to the ground.

In my early days as a doctor I had noticed that TB of the lungs, though it was a terrible disease, very often had the curious effect of making the sufferers more cheerful than is normal – perhaps it was a sort of euphoria. But Kirby Langford was not like that. He was as miserable as sin.

He had had a flourishing small business in Tonbridge called 'Three Lines', specializing in tea, coffee and spices. As his health deteriorated, he had taken his doctor's advice, sold up and retired to Winterham. 'Biggest mistake I ever made in my life,' he grumbled. 'Only got one line now, sitting on my backside.' I did point out gently that he was in no fit state to carry on his business, especially one involving lugging tea-chests around.

I asked him once if he had any outside interests. I knew there was a lively discussion group run by the vicar of Winterham quite nearby.

'What about the Vicar's discussion group?' I asked. I wasn't offering him the solace of religion when all else had failed, a sort of last-ditch succour for want of anything better, but I knew that it was the only way he would find meaning in an otherwise meaningless life.

'Religion!' said Kirby Langford, and he looked at me as if I had just crept out from under a stone. 'Religion! I had a belly-full of that at school – no thank you.'

After that, he still came to the surgery, but he usually picked the last possible moment before we closed the door so that he'd be the last to see me. I invited him to sit in one of Mrs Higginbotham's armchairs and occasionally she would give us a cup of tea while we chatted.

Then one day he came in with a speculative look in his eye. He was carrying the blue-covered Gideon's Bible which always lay on the waiting-room table.

'See this,' he waved the Bible at me. 'I've been reading it

in the waiting-room – you took a time with that last patient, didn't you? Well, I'm amazed – it really interested me. Could you get me one, in this version I mean?' I could and I did.

That winter the cold was too much for Kirby Langford even to walk to the surgery. So when I'd a free afternoon I'd drop in on him. He was full of questions about the things he was reading in his blue Bible.

I stopped there one afternoon and found him sitting in his chair by the fire. Some logs were spitting and blazing in the attractive old-fashioned open grate. He led off straightaway.

'I don't understand it, doc. Why didn't the clergymen who came to our school tell us what Jesus really said, instead of waffling on about religion in a vague sort of way?'

'I expect they were trying to, but you weren't on the right wavelength.'

'Yes, but look, it's straightforward enough. The question is, how does a bloke like me get started?'

'Pray.'

'What d'you mean – pray?'

'I mean, speak direct to Jesus. It may sound crazy, but he's there – it's not just imagination – and then he starts doing things. You'll see – things will change.'

'I don't see it, but OK, I'll have a go.'

When I called in next on Kirby Langford I found an extraordinary difference in him. It wasn't that he was any better physically, he was just holding his own. But it was the way he looked.

He hardly let me sit down before he began, 'I didn't really believe you, but see here, doc, it works! I didn't know how to begin your praying, so I just said whatever came into my head – and an extraordinary calm came over me. But there are things I must ask you. For instance,' he stabbed his finger into his blue-covered Bible, 'what does it really mean when Jesus talks about being forgiven? OK, I know if I forgive my Angela for not helping my wife I stop nagging her, but there must be more to it than that.'

It seemed a golden opportunity to try to explain the heart of Jesus' teaching to Kirby.

'When we deliberately do wrong, we put a block between

us and God . . . When Jesus sacrificed his life on the cross, he got rid of the block – so the way's clear to God. That's what forgiveness means. Don't ask me how it works, but it does.'

'Never saw it like that, but it sounds good sense. Thanks, doctor, you're a pal. Don't know how you put up with an old grumble-guts like me.'

Kirby Langford's general health still didn't improve. There was no miraculous healing. He stayed just the same, but he was a different man. He wasn't a pain in the neck to visit – he stopped moaning about his lot, and he lost his aggression.

I wasn't able to call on him as often as I might have wished, but I told the Winterham vicar about him and I heard they were getting on famously. I think the vicar, apart from giving Kirby Langford spiritual help, found he'd met his match at chess.

Attendances at the branch surgery continued to drop off so, at the end of the year, we closed it. I was glad, though, that we had had it for that year. I doubt if I would have got to know Kirby Langford otherwise.

13
Sea change

We woke around 6 a.m. Outside the wind was thrashing the trees. I switched on the bedside radio: '. . . English Channel: Dover, Wight, Portland, Plymouth, gale force 8 increasing storm force 10 – imminent'. I switched it off. That was more than enough.

'There was a twenty-four foot tide last night.' Elisabeth's nautical sense was working overtime.

I'm afraid we were both thinking, not about the safety of shipping in the Channel, but about our beach-hut. It was 'moored' insecurely to old logs which had been washed in by previous tides and hauled up the beach. The hut was just above normal high-water mark. Charles Semple, my senior partner, had had a half-share in it, but he'd given that up and it was our sole responsibility now. I wondered if he was awake and, if so, what he was feeling – probably great relief, I thought wryly!

Over the years since our arrival back from the remoteness of Africa, that lonely beach-hut had been, literally, a 'Godsend'. Not that we deserved it any more than anyone else. It was only a small affair, just a shack with a tarred felt roof, standing straight on the shingle.

Early on, when we first came to Wilverton, on rare occasions when we weren't too busy in the practice, we had picnicked with the children on a distant beach and we had seen there one or two huts, white and delightfully secluded, huddled together under the lee of a low, sloping chalk cliff.

Elisabeth had said longingly, 'Wouldn't it be fun if we owned one of those! We could just come and plonk ourselves down, make a cup of tea, change for a bathe and shelter in it if it turned nasty.' But we never thought the dream would come true.

Then a patient of ours, a garage-owner came in to see me one day. When the interview was over he said, 'You ought to be able to get away from us folk sometimes, doctor. Have you ever thought of a beach-hut? I've heard of an old customer of ours who's having to give up his. He used to be the harbour-master of Singapore, and he loved sitting in his hut looking at the sea. But he's not able to go down there now. Going cheap it is, only fifty quid.'

I thanked him, but fifty quid was too much for me. However, I mentioned it to Charles, who loves sailing, and he said slowly, 'What about sharing – fifty-fifty?'

I got the name of the old harbour-master and we did a deal. Fifty pounds it was. We had to pay an annual levy for the site to the Wilverton Town Council as well, but that was only a few pounds.

We took possession. We had to unload a selection of anchors and winches and other paraphernalia which the old chap had collected. We gave them to local fishermen and iron merchants, provided they came and took them away. In the end we had a roomy hut to use as we wished. We installed a second-hand Calor gas stove, china from the kitchen-cupboard and some deck-chairs. We had to carry fresh water from a distant tap near the road on the far side of the cliff.

There was one item from the past which we kept – a huge old leather armchair on iron runners, rusted with the salty air, obviously beloved by the harbour-master. It was superbly comfortable to lounge in in the sunshine – that is, when the sun did shine. Elisabeth and I took turns when we could get the children out of it. They loved it too and called it 'Heffalump'.

When the pace of the practice got too hot and there was an hour or two to spare, we'd up stakes and head for the beach-hut. And there, there was no hassle, nothing but the shingle, the sand and the seabirds and the everlasting sound of the sea. We looked out from the open front of the hut and there it stretched, due south, on and on, all the way to France. For a brief spell we could sit or walk or fish or bathe or put out to sea in one of our cronky old craft without a care. It was as if Wilverton front with its cars and people, and the surgery with its patients, visits and crises were as far away as France.

'Is this just escapism?' I asked Elisabeth as we sat soaking up the afternoon sunshine one half-day, sitting in our faded deck-chairs with the sand hot between our toes.

She pondered a while so, as I often do, I answered myself.

'Maybe it's more a case of *reculer pour mieux sauter*.'

'What *are* you talking about?' said Elisabeth impatiently without opening her eyes.

'It's French for being a long jumper,' I said in a poorly-concealed superior tone. 'Drawing back to be able to jump better – that's what we're doing at this beach-hut.'

'Well, you're going to have to do some jumping now,' she said, taking a glance at her wrist-watch. 'Just in time to get me home before you go to surgery.'

I stopped maundering and came back to earth with a bump. Perhaps the beach-hut was a bit of real life after all. You imagine you've got a hidey-hole – a Shangri-La – but you haven't. There's no such thing this side of heaven.

As I put on my respectable trousers, I found myself humming, 'Christian, seek not yet repose'. But that sea coast certainly had something. Its emptiness rested the mind, calmed it down. The crying of the gulls was balm for ears which were usually full of the complaints and demands of daily living – but not always.

There was the day when, clad in an old pair of Kenya shorts, I was walking blissfully along carrying a shrimping-net over my shoulder down to the sea, when I was hailed.

'Doctor Hamilton, Coo-ee, Doctor Hamilton.'

I turned and approaching hotfoot over the warm sand was Mrs Hawtree. Now Mrs Hawtree has at least a dozen serious complaints (in her own mind) but is remarkably fit for fifty-five. Somewhat breathlessly she spoke.

'Oh, doctor, I'm so glad I saw you. I know you won't mind my bothering you. You wouldn't have your prescription book on you? I forgot to ask you yesterday for my indigestion pills in the surgery, and when I saw you just now I felt it would save me another journey there tomorrow. I was just walking

Pedro when I spotted you.' Her Pekinese was sniffing suspiciously at my bare feet.

'What a pity, I don't happen to have my prescription pad *or* my fountain pen with me, Mrs Hawtree. I'm *so* sorry. I'll have to see you tomorrow after all. Bye now, I hope you have a nice walk.' I headed for the ocean at a steady trot. . .

When I was at school in London our family lived at Sidcup in Kent, and I often went to tea there with the Wimbrels, parents of one of my school-friends. After going to Africa I lost touch with them for many years, until quite unexpectedly one day Mr Wimbrel rang me up at the surgery.

'Andrew,' he said, as if twenty years had never happened. 'We've just retired here as I've left the bank now. We would like you to be our doctor, if you will.'

'You're sure you don't mind being looked after by someone you knew as a boy?' I said.

'No, not at all. That was ages ago,' he answered.

It wasn't long before he rang again. 'Mrs Wimbrel's not feeling very well. Could you come and see her?'

I knocked at the door and waited. I was surprised when Mrs Wimbrel herself came to the door. After all, she was supposed to be ill.

'Why, Andrew,' she said, 'haven't you grown!'

As I last saw her when I was over twenty I thought this unlikely, so I was worried. She had a weird, fey look about her. Sadly, I soon discovered that she had developed pre-senile dementia, probably brought on by the move and exhaustion. With very mild sedation and care she improved, but I didn't feel that she would ever fully recover.

About a year after this, there was a panic call from Wimbrel. 'I've lost Emmy,' he said. 'She went to the shops this morning and she never came back.'

It was 12.45. He had rung up all the shops he could think of. She had been to none of them. I told him I would contact the police. They instituted a search but Emmy had completely vanished. Wimbrel spent a worried night on his own, but next day his daughter came to be with him.

I had promised to take Elisabeth to the beach-hut after

111

morning surgery, so I had a word with Mrs Banbury to tell her where I would be. I felt I was doing no good by hanging about, but I kept thinking of Mrs Wimbrel – in her state of mind, anything could have happened.

We were walking along the edge of the cliff to go down the steep path to the hut when we saw the door of the hut flapping in the wind. We had had it broken into once before and our hearts sank.

I scrambled down the cliff ahead of Elisabeth and approached the hut gingerly. From inside came a sort of sighing groan and I pulled the door back. There on the floor, covered with her coat, was Mrs Wimbrel. She looked amazingly well considering that she could have been there for at least twenty-four hours.

'Hullo, Andrew. You are just in time for tea. Have you brought any milk? There isn't any here.' I could see that she had used the stove and boiled a kettle for herself during the time she'd been there. We always left a spare container for water in case of emergencies.

Elisabeth helped me to sit her in a chair. I remembered the day that Mrs Wimbrel and her husband had been walking along the beach, had seen us in our hut and we'd given them tea. I suspected that yesterday in her wandering she had vaguely remembered this as she had meandered aimlessly along that same stretch of beach.

But how had she unlocked the padlock? The answer was that I probably hadn't locked it when we had been down the time before. We made her comfy, got the kettle on the boil and made her tea and shared our sandwiches with her. I asked Elisabeth to keep an eye on her and went as quickly as I could to the phone. Soon two Wilverton ambulance-men were carrying out one of their more unusual assignments. . .

'I'm going down to the beach-hut,' said Charles.

It was a blistering day, but by lunch-time the sky had darkened and soon a tremendous storm burst over Wilverton. There was a dazzling show of forked lightning which seemed

112

to shoot into the sea just off the coast with explosions of thunder.

'Poor Dr Semple,' I said to Mrs Banbury at afternoon surgery. 'He's having a rotten day off.'

Just at that moment Charles came in. 'What on earth have you come into the surgery for?' I asked.

He didn't give me one of his normal terse replies. I glanced at his face. He looked in a shocked state. At last he said, 'We were sheltering in the hut,' his voice sounded more strained than I had ever heard it. 'The storm came in off the sea. There was an enormous flash and an explosion just behind the hut – and a boy,' he hesitated, 'a boy with a bike on the cliff-top was struck by lightning. I tore up the cliff. He was badly burned, and he was stone dead – cardiac arrest. The police took him to hospital by ambulance. One minute we were just watching that awe-inspiring storm and the next . . . Lilian and I won't forget it.' No Shangri-La, I thought.

Perhaps because of this or maybe because of Charles's increasing preoccupation with golf as a relaxation – he'd been a scratch golfer in his Cambridge days – whatever it was, he and Lilian were never so keen on the hut after that and in time they handed it over to us. Eventually we were able to forget the tragedy and as the years passed, we got to love that hut more and more.

We might have been going happily to that same hut brewing tea, writing letters, having a friend down, if it had not been for that day when we woke up to the grim weather forecast.

'I'll nip down there, when I've got through visits,' I said to Elisabeth. 'Just to see if the old hut's OK.'

I stopped the car in the coast road from where we usually went down to the beach below the cliff. There was an old friend of mine, Jos Blagdon, the gipsy who had once rescued us when our caravan had broken down. Jos never misses a trick. His horse was tethered, cropping the short grass on the cliff-top and his cart was just off the road. He was loading it with lumber, boards, lengths of timber and logs – most of it broken but some intact.

'What's all this, Jos?' I asked.

'Want ter see what's dahn there!' he said, jerking his thumb towards the cliff-path. I didn't wait for more. As I got to the cliff edge I stared down. All that was left of the group of huts below were some piles of shattered painted wood. Of our hut nothing remained – nothing at all. No, I was wrong – as I went down the path, I saw our heavy Calor gas cylinder lying at an angle, half-buried in sand and shingle – but no hut, not a trace. And Heffalump – Heffalump had gone with the rest. It seemed like a bereavement.

When Barney came home from school for the holidays, he went down to the beach on his bicycle to inspect the damage. That night when we were having supper he suddenly said, 'Dad, honestly, I'm surprised at you. Fancy letting this get you down. I bet we could build another hut.'

He was right. We found the names of the other owners whose huts had been demolished in the gale and we bought one of the wrecks for a song; we were also given the remains of several other huts for nothing. Most people had given up all hope of ever having a site on the beach again.

Barney and I – mostly Barney – put together a very respectable hut. It was a bit tatty in places, but in many ways it was better than the one we'd had before. We even got a dinghy from one of the people who had given up their hut, so we could get afloat again too. At last we had it ready – but not until the end of September.

Elisabeth and I were sitting one afternoon on even more second-hand deck-chairs and she was looking at the Channel shipping through some old field-glasses. It was an enormous spring tide and the sea was farther out than we had ever seen it.

'Andy,' she said suddenly. '*Look*!'

I looked through the glasses where she was pointing. I couldn't see anything unusual at first; then I spotted it, poised in a crevice of the rocks, way beyond the normal low tidemark. It was Heffalump, looking as if he were waiting for Neptune himself to take his seat.

We rushed down the beach before the tide turned, and wrenched and levered our old friend free and carried him up to the hut in triumph.

It was still Heffalump, but he would never be quite the same. He was in need of total renovation. Seaweed had grown on him, sand had filled any available openings and his leather cover was a sodden remnant. He had suffered a sea change but – we intended to rehabilitate him and put him to good use once more. . .

Spring had come round again and we had snatched an afternoon not long after Easter to pop down to the hut. We were sitting in the open doorway with a low-lying sun streaming in. Suddenly, and *à propos* of apparently nothing in particular, Elisabeth said, 'I am the resurrection and the life.'

For a moment I was nonplussed. She is not given to outbursts of fervour. Then I understood what had inspired her, curled up there in a newly-covered Heffalump. She was thinking of the arrival of spring, of an old lady rescued from disaster, of a boy lying dead on the cliff-top and of our hut, destroyed in the gale and now rebuilt. They had reminded her, in an odd sort of a way, of those incomparable words of Jesus Christ.

14

The hidden menace

Wearily I lifted my head and looked at the clock. It was slightly out of focus. I was beginning to feel really fed up with reading those pages and pages of close print and it was getting late. At that moment Elisabeth came in holding a large cup of steaming tea.

'Here you are, love, you look as if you need it. But isn't it time you packed it in and came to bed? It's a quarter to twelve and I won't sleep till you come.'

'I know,' I said irritably, 'but I've got to find it. I know it's here somewhere.' I sipped the tea gratefully.

Elisabeth sat down in her dressing-down in front of the fire. The red glow from the embers lit up her face. I forgot what I was looking for for the moment as I realized how much I loved that profile. Nose a bit long perhaps, but so straight, and those big, kind eyes. Her dressing-gown was faded and neatly patched down one side. She is awful about spending money on herself. I sighed, thinking how grateful I was that she wasn't the sort of wife who ruined her husband with extravagant shopping sprees for new outfits.

She got up and quietly went off to bed to wait for me to come.

I turned back to the sheaf of papers in the folder on the table. I knew the answer was there somewhere. I just knew it. The cover had the title 'Toxic Chemicals used in Industry'. Not very exciting. It had been Fred, my partner, who had suggested that the BMA Library might be able to help in my problem. So I had written to them and they'd sent this tome I was now wading through.

I looked again at the index and ran my finger down the list of lethal substances used in modern manufacturing processes. That was it – must be it! That was the name that had rung bells when I was reading through the text: 'Isocyanates'. I flipped over the references listed in the index.

'Involved in the manufacture and application of new forms of resin paints. Used in the hardening process.'

It had got to be the answer. I wrote some notes on a pad, shut the file and went to bed.

The start of the whole business had been when Bruce Featherstone's wife called me to see him in their little semi-detached on the outskirts of Wilverton. Bruce had been on our list for years. His record-card showed that he was the ideal patient: he brought in his National Health Service annual pound or two and never bothered us!

Phyl Featherstone greeted me.

'I don't know what's come over Bruce. He's never ill, but over the past few days he's been very different – puffing and blowing and wheezing when he comes home from work. Today I really think he's got bronchitis'. Phyllis worked part-time in a chemist's shop so she was used to seeing people collecting prescriptions for chest trouble.

'Hullo, stranger,' said Bruce trying to sound cheerful as I walked into the bedroom.

I didn't like the look of him at all. His complexion was quite bluish and he was breathing like a broken-down cab-horse. When I had examined him I was still puzzled.

'You've got bronchitis and asthma, Bruce. What have you been doing?'

'Nothing, doc – just my job. I'm a paint-sprayer at Briggs. You knew I worked for them, didn't you?

Briggs Bros was the biggest industrial concern in Wilverton. There aren't many – Wilverton survives mainly on holiday visitors and its small fishing industry. They were a good enough company. But when Bruce said 'paint-spraying', a faint warning-bell sounded in my mind.

'Never given me any trouble before,' he went on. 'Been doing the job for years. We've just started using a marvellous new stuff, wouldn't mind getting it on my old jalopy – a resin paint. Once it's on, never wears off – or so they say.'

I gave him antibiotics and tablets to open up his bronchial passages – and a sick certificate.

A week later he was as right as rain. Perhaps I should have been clever enough to foresee what was going to happen. Bruce hadn't been back at work two days before he was ill again with exactly the same symptoms as before.

That's when I smelled a rat. It had to be something at work that was causing his chest trouble. I talked it over with Fred, and that was when he suggested contacting the BMA Reference Library.

After my late-night session poring over industrial poisons, I asked Mrs Banbury at the end of the next morning's surgery to get me the manager of Briggs Bros on the phone if he were available.

She put him through.

We exchanged a few pleasantries. I knew him vaguely – a rather suave, go-getter who might cut corners.

'Could you tell me anything about the chemicals involved in your new paint-spraying process?' I asked.

I sensed a guardedness in his voice as he answered, 'Certainly, but why do you want to know?'

'Simply that a patient of mine who works for you might be allergic to one of them.'

When he spoked again, his voice was cold and clipped. He reeled off a list of names in which that malign substance 'Isocyanates' cropped up again.

'I can assure you, doctor,' he was very formal now, 'that we take all the prescribed precautions to safeguard the health of our working personnel, to obviate any risks. You can come and see for yourself if you wish.'

'Thank you very much. I may do just that. I am sorry to have disturbed you. Goodbye.' I sat and thought, 'This is too hot a potato for me to handle by myself.'

Fred came up with more good advice. 'There's an official body called the Health and Safety Executive. Why don't you get in touch with them?'

I did. It was arranged for Dr Crabtree, one of their staff, to come with me to the factory the following Friday.

The foreman had been detailed to show us round. All was in apple-pie order – including the paint-spraying bay, complete with water channel to absorb noxious vapours, extractor fans, positive pressure-masks for workmen, the lot.

We thanked the foreman and left the building.

'Seems OK,' said Crabtree. 'Nothing to fault there. Are you sure that your patient hasn't a tendency to bronchitis anyway?'

'Never to my knowledge,' I replied.

As we were walking through the gate to my car, a man in overalls with a lunch-box in his hand slouched forward.

'Are you the docs what's been inspecting the works?' he queried. ''Eard about you – all round the works it is. Do you want to know somethin'? I bet you never found nothin' wrong, did you? Course you didn't – all laid on for you wasn't it? Well, I'll tell you – it ain't like that always. 'Arf the time them fans don't work, and the gas-masks are only used when the factory inspector comes round. The men couldn't do the job in the time given if they wore 'em. I'll say cheerio then. Don't tell anyone I told you or I'll get the sack.' He glanced around cautiously and meandered back into the works.

'Phew!' I said. 'That alters the picture a bit.'

'I'm afraid it isn't as simple as all that,' said Crabtree, frowning as we got into my car. 'How do we prove it – on the word of a workman who's scared of losing his job? You'll have to do better than that. You don't even know for certain that your patient is adversely affected by isocyanates.' I felt resentful that he couldn't take action, but I had to see his point.

Bruce Featherstone resigned his job off his own bat and I reconciled myself to defeat when he completely recovered in a further two weeks. He got no compensation from the firm because he'd done the resigning. I heard he was trying his hand in a totally different occupation – working on a farm.

I was returning one day from visiting one of our outlying patients when I remembered Bruce. His new employers farmed just down the down. It wouldn't take more than a few minutes out of the day to drop in on the farm and I could find out how he was getting on.

As I moved down the narrow lane I saw that over the

hedge a red tractor was approaching in the field. It was towing a loaded farm truck. Suddenly, to my horror, I realized that the driver was engaged in muck-spreading. There was no escape. I halted the car. On thundered the tractor, its drive-shaft turning a whirling apparatus like the spokes of a giant umbrella. Dung flew in a huge arc behind it. Over the field it went and over the hedge, and as he passed me, over the car. I closed the window just in time as lumps of extremely fruity cow-dung rained down.

As he passed, the driver saw what had happened and stopped just beyond me, jumped out of his cab and walked round to peer over the hedge at my vehicle deluged in dung. Through the bespattered window I recognized Bruce. As a new hand, he had obviously not realized the field of fire of his machine.

I couldn't be angry – the situation reminded me ludicrously of the hippopotami of Africa who mark their territory by trotting round the borders, performing as they go and using their stumpy tails in exactly the manner of Bruce's muck-spreader. When I managed to stop laughing, I opened the door.

'Hullo, Bruce. Is that the way you treat your doctor?'

'I'm right sorry,' he said. 'Never saw you coming. Here, I'll clear it off.' He took a wisp of hay from the field. Finding a gate, he climbed into the lane and began clearing his boss's best cow-manure from the car.

He had never felt fitter in his life, he told me. So far as he was concerned, bronchitis and isocyanates and Briggs Bros belonged to a past he wanted to forget. It seemed I had better fall in line too.

And so the case would have rested if James Cragg had not turned up some weeks later to see me – complaining of wheezing and bronchitis. True, he had had a little trouble that way before, but he'd been well for years.

After examining him I asked, 'What's your job?'

'I work on a moulding machine making plastic components for export.'

'Who's your employer?'

'Briggs Bros.'

My nostrils twitched. 'What's the plastic made with?'

'A sort of resin which needs a hardener.'

I signed him off work. That night I consulted my folder on industrial toxins again. I found it under 'resins'. There was the word again: 'Isocyanate – can give rise to asthma-like symptoms, either through direct irritation of the bronchioles or by an allergic mechanism.'

I still had insufficient evidence to work on. But a week later Cragg went back to work and two days afterwards he was on his sick-bed again, this time really fighting for his breath.

Between gasps he answered my questions as best he could. No, they did not wear masks while working – there were no masks. Yes, there were fumes – they stuck in your throat.

I made an appointment for Cragg at a London chest hospital. When he was well enough, he went by train armed with my letter.

Three weeks later I had the hospital's report: 'the patient suffers from a condition of broncho-spasm induced by a reaction to isocyanate. He should never work in contact with these substances again.'

Through the Health and Safety Executive I obtained an instruction to Briggs Bros that they should immediately install safety procedures in their plastic moulding shop.

Unfortunately, James Cragg did not fare as well as Bruce Featherstone. His health did not improve and for months he was so badly affected that it seemed doubtful whether he would ever be able to work again.

But he was also of a different temperament from Featherstone. He wasn't going to take this lying down. He saw a solicitor and aimed to sue Briggs for negligence. In not providing adequate precautions for workers in the plastic moulding works, he claimed that they were responsible for his damaged health, his inability to perform any heavy work in the future, and his loss of wages.

Briggs denied responsibility and I understood that the solicitor briefed Enslicott, the Middle Temple barrister from Wilverton to act for Cragg. Enslicott's medico-legal expertise would prove invaluable, I felt sure. For my part, I wrote full reports for Cragg. The chest hospital also submitted reports. Then Briggs' insurance company instructed a London solicitor, who contacted me for my surrender of my medical records. I did this quite gladly, they would do them no good whatsoever.

Eventually, with an action in the High Court pending, the matter was settled out of court. Cragg was awarded £27,000 damages against Briggs Bros.

I tried not to feel exultant at Briggs Bros getting their come-uppance–but they had asked for it. No further case of isocyanate poisoning has ever come my way again.

15

The surgeon
and the Salvationist

MacFarlane was our senior local general surgeon and his skill
was called on for everything from varicose veins to breast
cancer. He looked older than his fifty years, but I knew he
was fitter than most men of his age. Nothing stopped him
going on his early morning run before he got down to his
arduous round of duties. He'd recently taken part with
fellows less than half his age, in a charity walk from
Wilverton to Brighton.

He always dressed in baggy Harris tweed suits although
he must have had a good salary. I reckon surgeons earn every
penny they are paid. Reimbursement for the tension and
sheer mental and physical stress under which they work is
beyond computation. No one holds the surgeon's hand, yet
he holds the patient's life in his.

Perhaps that's a statement that needs modification. In the
mission hospital where I used to work in the East End of
London, there is a text inscribed on the wall of the operating
theatre, just where it will catch the surgeon's eye, when he
lifts it from the patient for a moment. It reads, 'I, the Lord,
will hold thy right hand.' 'Pity', McNeill-Love, the honorary
surgeon, used to say, 'I'm left-handed.'

I followed MacFarlane down the stairs and he half-turned,
compressed his lips and shook his greying head. He had come
in response to my request for an emergency consultation over
an elderly patient of mine who had suddenly collapsed in
shock and severe abdominal pain. I had had the call just as
I was beginning lunch.

I found old Mr Fenton curled up on a sofa with his housekeeper hovering anxiously over him. He was pale and sweat-
ing and he managed to gasp, between groans, 'There's a

terrible pain here.' He spread his hands all over his tummy. 'Do something to help me, doctor.'

After a quick examination I gave him an injection of morphine and rang up MacFarlane. 'I think this chap has got a mesenteric thrombosis, but I would like your opinion before admitting him.' Because of the special nature of the symptoms this seemed to me the likeliest diagnosis – the blocking of a blood vessel supplying the intestine.

In the dining-room downstairs, MacFarlane shook his head again.

'No, not a thrombosed mesenteric, Hamilton, he's too bad for that. He's got a dissecting aneurism of the aorta, unless I'm ver-r-ra much mistaken.' I noticed he always rolls his 'r's' when he's very serious. 'It would simply be cruelty to take him to the hospital. He will be dead within the hour.'

How could MacFarlane be so sure?

Forty-five minutes later, freed from pain by the morphine, Mr Fenton slipped quietly away. I said a prayer with the housekeeper as she sat by her old employer, her face in her hands, while the tears trickled between her fingers. From the study, I made all the arrangements for a post-mortem. When I got home I found Elisabeth had put my lunch in the oven for me. It's true that the life of a doctor hardens you, but somehow I wasn't feeling hungry any more.

In three days I got the pathologist's post-mortem report: 'Massive dissecting aortic aneurism.' The wall of the main abdominal artery was split along its length and filled with blood clot. Absolutely nothing could have been done. I simply had to admire the pin-point accuracy of MacFarlane's diagnosis and advice. So many diagnoses were possible in a man of eighty-two, but he had been absolutely right.

With MacFarlane it was a mixture of observation and experience – and something else. Genius? Instinct? Call it what you will – he'd got it. Mind you, some people called him a crank and some just said he was dour, and he certainly did have some personal fads. He believed in masses of fibre in the diet – something research has now amply confirmed as being beneficial. He also treated leg ulcers with honey.

Recently I had got to know him quite well and called him frequently when I needed a second opinion.

I was still surprised and honoured when I met him one day, after a visit made on the edge of Wilverton, and he said, 'Got a minute? I'd like to show ye something.' But it wasn't at all what I expected.

There was a stretch of land devoted to allotments which lay just beyond the edge of the housing estate we were in. MacFarlane led me down a passage between the houses and out into it. We walked past flourishing plots dotted with little sheds and butts of water to a big area on the far side. This was his. Giant cauliflowers, runner-beans, cabbages, and beetroot were growing here and amongst many other vegetables, there was even a long mound of asparagus, now in the foliage stage.

'This is how I keep fit,' he grinned. 'Growing *and* eating what I grow!' He even had several beehives along the edge of the plot. It began to look as if he had a vested interest in some of his own treatments.

'I keep a pig in the shed at the bottom of my garden too. Feed him mostly on veg I canna use and on neighbour's scraps – use very little meal. He supplies manure for the plot in return.'

We walked slowly back towards my car. He went on talking through the window as I got in to continue my round.

'My wife died some years back, you know, and the boys are all away now. But I've found a new family – the lads in the youth fellowship at our Presbyterian kirk. Och, they're a great bunch. We skelped the Salvationists the other day at fitba.' In his enthusiasm he was lapsing more and more into his native Glaswegian. 'Ah, an' there's a graund wee body that organizes them, a *woman*, ye ken. Ye must meet her, Hamilton. I'm aye meetin' her on committees mesel'.'

So Elisabeth and I found ourselves having tea with MacFarlane in his untidy but comfortable lounge and meeting Mrs Farthing, the Salvationist who ran the boys' club for the 'Army'. It was a most ecumenical tea-party. The Kirk, the Salvation Army and the Church of England all together and finding common ground in the Bible. As

125

MacFarlane put it, 'It's no' the bonnet ye're wearin' but the road ye're treadin' that matters.'

It wasn't such a surprise when, a week later, I had an invitation from Mrs Farthing to come to her house to help in a discussion group she had founded in addition to her work with the youth club.

'I think a lot of them are communists,' she enlightened me. 'There are one or two from my husband's factory. He works for an old-established firm of rope-makers. They've existed in Wilverton since it had a fleet of fishing luggers, but now he makes nylon ropes for racing yachts.'

I wasn't quite sure how I qualified as a guest of honour at a communist get-together – probably as an Aunt Sally, I thought.

On the very evening I promised to go I had a late call to see Tommy Bernstein. He and I were great pals. When I first went to see him when he was about four, for 'bronchial chest', he seemed a bit shy of me, and had hidden under the bed-clothes. I bribed him to come out by offering him the use of my 'telephone' – stethoscope to anyone else. He really enjoyed carrying on a conversation with me whispering into the ear-pieces.

His condition now puzzled and worried me. He had a moderate temperature and his mother said she had thought that he had had 'flu for the past three to four days but should now be getting better.

I asked, 'Anything else you've noticed?'

'Well, it's an odd thing, doctor, he's drinking such a lot. See that jug? He's emptied that five times today already. Of course, he's in and out of the toilet all the time as well. I wouldn't have thought he was all that feverish.'

I began to be suspicious.

'Mrs Bernstein, could you get him to pass some water in a jar for me?'

I tested his urine with one of the sensitive strips I carry in a bottle and there it was – sugar. It might just be a rare occurrence – he could be a child with a low kidney threshold: the blood sugar is still quite normal and spills over to the urine because, as it were, the barrier is lower than normal.

126

But I guessed this wasn't the case with Tommy. I was afraid he had become a diabetic.

I went downstairs with his mother. The prospect of life-long injections of insulin, plus a special diet and so forth for their own child can be very frightening to a parent, but it had to be considered.

'Are there any relatives whom you know who had trouble with too much sugar in their system, Mrs Bernstein?'

'Well, his grandfather on his dad's side was diabetic – oh, you don't think that Tommy is diabetic, do you, doctor?'

I spoke in a matter-of-fact voice. 'Well, there is a chance that he is, I'm afraid, but don't let's cross all the bridges before we get to them. I would like him in the children's ward at the hospital for assessment.'

'Tonight, doctor?'

'Yes, I think so – the sooner he's there, the sooner we will know.'

We arranged his admission on the telephone and I told Tommy what a good time children had on the ward. He seemed to be almost looking forward to it!

I'd been there half an hour and now I was going to be late for Mrs Farthing's evening with the communists. I apologized as she opened the door and she led me into the front room.

The atmosphere was pretty heavy. Around the wall on the sofa and dining-room chairs sat about eight men. They were of varying ages but mostly young. I knew some of them by sight; there was Bert who was a council road-digger, Graham from the wood-yard in town, Kevin who was a milk roundsman. There were other faces I didn't recognize.

Mrs Farthing introduced me. 'This is Doctor Hamilton, I told you I was asking him along. I'll go and make some tea.' She fled.

They were looking at me with a mixture of interest and resentment, but some seemed quite friendly.

'Evening, all,' I sounded just like Dixon of Dock Green.

'Evening,' was their partial response.

Better take the plunge. 'I'm not quite sure why I'm here, but I understand you're discussing politics and Mrs Farthing thought you might be interested in the way I look at things. Would I be right in guessing that most of you would call yourself communists?'

'Too right you would, doctor,' a rather hard-faced man replied, who was sitting over by the fire.

'OK, so you expect me to form the opposition? Bit tough on me – one against eight, but I don't see it like that. I'm not here as a member of the middle-class establishment to try and change your views.'

'Couldn't if you tried,' came from the man by the fireplace.

I decided to stick my neck out and not get involved in endless arguments. 'I could say what I think – that would be just my ideas and you are entitled to yours, so we might not get very far. Wouldn't it be better to take an independent view and see what the Bible says?'

'Blimey, a religious nut.' It was the man by the fireplace again. 'See 'ere, doctor, we're communists right?'

'Why?'

'Because we see it's the only way to get social justice, and a decent wage for working blokes like us.' There was a murmur of assent around the room.

'I couldn't agree more,' I said. 'But you'd be surprised what the Bible says about it. How about this?' I took a paperback New Testament out of my pocket. It was a modern version I had just received from a friend in America. I turned the pages to James chapter five and read aloud:

' "Now, you rich people, listen to me; weep and wail over the miseries that are coming upon you; your riches have rotted away. You have piled them up against these last days. You've not paid the wages to the men who worked your fields. Listen to their complaints. The cries of those who labour in your fields have reached the ears of God." '

The fireplace man put out his hand. 'Is that in the Bible?' I gave him the book and he scanned it with a comical look of sheer disbelief.

I took my chance and continued. 'The Bible shows us that we should love one another. You do believe that, don't you? Well, we can't love one another unless we love God first!'

I don't know how much we achieved that evening but I

know that before the meeting ended we were discussing whether it was possible to change human nature, and we'd even begun to consider whether only Jesus could do that and what the meaning of his death on the cross was.

I think Mrs Farthing had been listening at the door. Her eyes were sparkling as she came in with a tray of steaming mugs of tea.

I had to go soon after that, although it looked as if they were ready to stay all night talking. "Night, doc,' said the fireplace man and stuck out his hairy hand. 'Come again.'

I did – several times over the next few months, and I learned a lot. The group of us became real friends. Bert, the road-digger, gave me a thumbs-up one day when I passed him on my way to visit a patient and another day told me where I could get cheap fertilizer for the garden by joining the Allotment Association for a small fee, even though my allotment was just my own garden.

I met Mrs Farthing in the supermarket when I was picking up some bargain margarine Elisabeth had spotted in *The Wilverton Advertiser*.

'I know you won't believe it, doctor,' she said, 'but Mr Kingsbury, that man by the fireplace who came the first night we had a discussion – well he's joined the Army and even belongs to the men's Bible Study *and* he's playing the cornet in the band!'

16
One down
and two to go

We sat there exhausted, Elisabeth and I, relaxing in the warm evening sun at the open end of the marquee. We were in that state, not wholly unpleasant, of maudlin sentimentality, induced, not by alcohol for, true to our obstinate convictions, there had been nothing stronger at the reception than apple juice. One or two of the guests might have been a little disappointed but, there it was; even Sarah hadn't wanted it, and, after all, it was her wedding.

Up at the other end of the marquee Peter and Barney, still resplendent in their morning suits, were ostensibly 'clearing up'. They were certainly clearing up the salmon and cucumber sandwiches, but they did deserve a bit of nourishment; it had been all go, right up to the departure of the last guest. One of the suits had been hired; we hoped Peter wasn't getting it mucked up. The other was a family heirloom from my father, made by a London tailor.

'It was a lovely service.' Elisabeth's eyes were misty.

'Pity young Hargreaves chose the photograph session to throw a "hypo". I thought he'd learnt to manage his insulin by now. Must have been the excitement,' I muttered.

'It was a good job Barney spotted him,' said Elisabeth. 'He just dropped down behind the crowd. Good thing there were those sugar lumps in the vestry too, to bring him round!'

'Well, Barney's medical education's not cheap, we deserve a bit of return. I do wish he'd concentrate a bit more on the medical books though; seems he spends half his time reading philosophy and attending to down-and-outs.

'Now you know perfectly well that Barney's got through all his exams so far. It's just that he's interested in people,

130

not only illnesses.' Elisabeth sprang to the defence of our youngest.

'I thought Sarah looked wonderful in that cream satin,' she went on dreamily.

'She should have done, it cost enough!' I said, but I thought she had too. She was a tall girl, half a head taller than Elisabeth, but she had the same wide-apart greeny-brown eyes. She had a determined chin too, but I suppose she got that from me. It was a good job that the auburn-haired young man who had today removed her from our family circle was even taller than she – it wouldn't have done for her to be able to look down on her husband.

David was an old school-friend of Peter's. We'd guessed something was up when Sarah had found it essential for her studies to go over to his father's farm with great frequency because of the unique geological features of the district, even though she *was* doing geology as one of her subjects at Keele University. She was keen, but not *that* keen.

'He's asked me to marry him,' she'd announced when she came home for the last vacation before taking her degree. 'It's all right, I'd already decided I was going to. The only thing that worried me was – could he cope with dad?'

'Well! Of all the . . .' I stopped. I supposed that after all these years of bossing patients around perhaps I had become a mite domineering. But – David didn't seem to mind me too much. He laughed at all my jokes, which is a fair test of anyone's stamina.

'Which reminds me,' I said to Elisabeth, who hadn't the faintest idea of what had been going through my mind, 'that was a good story that David's brother told.'

'What, about Buttercup Joe?' Elisabeth smiled.

It had all been so unexpected. Frank had seemed such a quiet young man, so different from David, who was full of fun. He was supposed to be proposing the health of the bridesmaids too, in his speech. They did get a mention at the end, but only just. He had risen to his feet, rapped the table and begun:

'Ladies and gentlemen, as brother of the bridegroom, I find myself in a position of some delicacy.' There had followed some outrageous revelations about David for which I was sure Frank would pay dearly later, and then he told us the tale of Buttercup Joe – in a faultless West Country accent.

'It were loike this yere: parson, 'e were a traipsin' 'ome one noight after choir pra-actice when 'oo should 'e meet but 'ole Buttercup Joe a'bearin' a la-antern in 'is 'a-and.

' "Hello, Joe," sez parson, friendly-loike, "And where are you going to, my good man?"

"Parson, oi be goin' a courtin'."

"But Joe, when I went courting, I never took a lantern."

". . . Ar, parson-and look wot you got!" '

There was a rapturous response to his tale, far more than I was later accorded for my disclosures of Sarah's early days.

It seemed the season for banalities.

'Well, that's the first one gone. Good job we haven't any more daughters – nuptials come expensive these days.'

Elisabeth was gazing fixedly through the opening of the marquee door at the distant outline of the Downs, shadowy against the skyline. 'Do you think we've failed them? Not given them firm enough guide-lines? . . . Mind you, I don't agree with that chap at the medical conference you took me to, going on about shielding your children from adverse influences while giving them freedom of expression – didn't seem to work very well with his children, did it? D'you remember them at lunch? They had freedom of expression, all right, throwing food about – *and* he shielded them from adverse influences! Remember that manageress hovering round their table? She was an adverse influence if ever I saw one!' Elisabeth has quite a sharp wit for all her demure appearance.

She'd got me going though. Weddings are a season for reviewing the past and indeed some of it didn't look all that rosy. Even Barney had got one below the belt after the ceremony. I was having a bit of an argument with Elisabeth over placings in the photographs and he slyly whispered, 'Dad, you promised to cherish Mum at *your* wedding. How about it?'

Sitting there with it all over, it was only too easy to think

132

of past failures. I remembered when Barney himself had woken me, when he was quite small, yelling his head off for nothing in particular, and I'd had a series of bad nights on call and Elisabeth was just recovering from an operation. I'd smacked him, hard. I was often getting health visitors and social workers to call on parents I suspected of baby-battering. Lucky I wasn't up before the court myself then.

Oh well, I suppose they hadn't turned out too badly, though perhaps I'd been responsible for infecting them all for better or worse with the games bug. I remembered Pete, carried off the field twice at rugger: once at school, when he split his lip clean through on the opposing scrum-half's head and had six stitches; then at his agricultural college, getting concussion – the trouble was, he would lead with his head! That put a stop to his rugger, being in bed for a week. His team-mates had been very kind – especially as they knew he didn't get tight with them; in fact, he often baled them out of pubs when trouble began. They kept coming to his room to ask how 'the vicar' was!

Sarah had been almost as bad. Unfortunately she took to discus-throwing on top of everything else. That ghastly occasion of the school athletic sports came back to me vividly. My medical skill was so nearly called upon. All the parents were gathering round the trestle-table for tea when Sarah threw her first discus. Unfortunately its trajectory was at right angles to its appointed path. 'Oh! Look out!' screamed the headmistress, just in time, as the discus landed and took away a trestle, precipitating bread and butter, cakes, bowls of strawberries and cream and cups of tea on to the grass beneath.

Barney was the most sedate in his sporting tendencies merely playing hockey for the United Hospitals when he remembered to turn up.

I suppose, if anyone had bothered to ask us, I'd have said that we'd had only a few ideas that we'd tried to follow in bringing them up, and we'd stuck to those. Being consistent and backing each other up; apologizing – especially to the children – if we got it wrong; trying to make a regular habit of praying and reading the Bible as a family *and* of having

133

fun together; taking our hands off and letting go . . . and now, Sarah had gone. . .

The telephone went in the house. Mrs Clout came down the steps. 'Doctor,' she called, 'It's Mrs Banbury from the surgery.'

'I'm so sorry to bother you, doctor, but it's Johnny Taggerty's mother, she especially wanted you. Johnny's very bad. She says he keeps talking about the doctor from the 'house Jack built', says you'll know what he means. Do you think you could possibly see him? Is the reception over?'

'Not to worry, Mrs Banbury, I'll go. It'll get me out of the clearing up.'

17

A door in the wall

'Fred, are you thinking of going to the GP lecture at Hollin-bourne on Saturday? It's dealing with marital disharmony. There's a couple of psychiatrists talking, and the resident Senior Medical Officer.'

'Yes, I had thought about it.'

'Well, would you like to come in my new bus? I want to do a bit of mileage to help run it in.'

'Right – provided you drive carefully!'

The car was a VW Varient. I was going to enjoy showing it off. At least, that was the idea. But the usual Volkswagen snarl was a mere coughing grumble and I had to change down even on the slightest incline.

'What's the matter with it?' Fred looked across at me.

'Don't know,' I said, feeling rather irritated. 'But it's going back to the garage on Monday.'

The man who gave the main lecture was impressive – in appearance, that is. He was an American with a bushy black beard which covered most of his face and large, horn-rimmed glasses covering the rest. He talked for three-quarters of an hour, mostly in psychiatrist's jargon which was about as revealing as his beard.

Then, right at the end of his lecture, he produced a real gem of clear common sense, which everyone understood, even me.

'If a husband and wife become estranged and they have built up a wall between them, it's no good trying to break down the whole structure at once. You've got to help them find one tiny little door through to each other. It could be she hates your British steak and kidney pudding – an' I don't blame her – but that's his favourite all the same. Suppose she's willing to cook it for him just one night a week? Then, instead of the husband going out every night to the local bar, suppose he stays home one night and they watch television together. It could be, just through a little opening like that, that reconciliation can begin to take place.'

I could see that this idea applied to more than just marital breakdown, and I was still dwelling on it on Monday morning when the garage man discovered that they'd left off a plug-lead on the Varient. Of course, I could have found that myself, but I'm no mechanic. I let the manager know I wasn't impressed with their pre-delivery check up.

As I drove away with the engine snarling nicely, I began going over the lecturer's idea again. It reminded me of the children's story, *The Secret Garden*, and the little girl who unlocks a door in the garden wall to discover a whole new world the other side. At lunch-time, I shared my musings with Elisabeth.

'We're all building walls, all the time, aren't we?' I said. 'We shut other people out of our lives or we hide behind defensive walls or else we just find ourselves hemmed in by walls, like the fear of illness. And what about walls dividing races, husbands and wives, parents and children, classes . . . It's often left to us doctors to help people find a way through,' I concluded rather pompously.

It wasn't long afterwards that I discovered I'd built a little wall of my own. . .

'You aren't going to like this,' said Mrs Banbury.

'Not Miss Andrews?' I groaned, looking into the visiting book.

''Fraid so,' said Mrs Banbury. 'She simply *must* see you today.'

'But I only saw her last week.'

'Sorry, but she won't take no for an answer.'

I had recently calculated that the said lady had asked for visits 200 times in the last five years, mostly for illnesses she had just thought up or read about in her well-thumbed copy of *The Home Doctor*. I had for some time been aware that she would always be sitting in the bay-window of her flat, waiting for my car to approach. By the time I had got out, climbed the short flight of stairs to the front door, knocked and entered her room, she would be in bed, clothes pulled up to her chin, eyes shut, and apparently needing to be aroused from an exhausted stupor.

Well, this time I wasn't going to play ball. I decided on a stratagem. I stopped the car around the corner, walked under cover of the wall along the front of the gardens, tore up the steps and walked straight into her room. She had barely risen from the chair in the window.

'Hullo, Miss Andrews,' I said, smiling grimly. 'So glad to find you better today and able to be up and about.' It was my shortest visit ever and I congratulated myself on the success of my ploy as I went down the steps.

But – I wasn't feeling very happy, I wasn't feeling happy at all. I sat in the front of the car and thought. What had my little trick achieved? Did I really know Miss Andrews? In all these years, had I ever really troubled to find out why she was always sending for the doctor? I'd just put up with it – with a bad grace.

Once she'd even rung from a neighbour's flat and asked, in an assumed voice, for a visit 'for my neighbour Miss Andrews'. I've no doubt that the neighbour had finally jibbed at making unnecessary calls for her, and made her phone herself. But I'd recognized her voice; had I ever recognized the one inside trying vainly to be heard? No, I'd built up a nice defensive wall in my mind to keep her out so that I could not hear.

I got out of the car and walked back into the flat. Miss Andrews was sitting on the edge of her bed, crying. I sat down beside her and put an arm round her shoulders. It took some time but in the end she haltingly told me some of the things I wanted to know.

She was a country girl, it turned out. Her father had been bailiff on a large estate in Hertfordshire and her youngest brother had been a gamekeeper there. She'd felt secure and happy in that home. Then her brother had been called up for the Hitler war and was killed in France. Her father died shortly afterwards. Years of caring for her mother followed and then, finally, she was left, completely alone. So she had moved south.

It was perfectly obvious that she needed a man in her life, but it was too late for her to get a husband. The next best thing had been for her to care for an old retired seaman who lived in the flat above, but, before long, he had had to go permanently into hospital and so she was once again quite alone.

Though she only subconsciously realized it, she had been asking for doctors' visits simply to have a man call in. Then, that very day, her ancient radio had packed up and, as if that wasn't enough, I had brutally exposed her little charade. It had been the last straw. Telling me didn't solve all her problems but at least it helped her to do it.

What really helped was when my wireless-expert friend, Buttercup Joe, agreed to call in on her and fix her set. He developed the habit of dropping in at regular intervals, 'just to see it was working all right', and he would often stop for a cup of tea and a chat into the bargain.

Calls from Miss Andrews became a rarity. In fact, if I was in the vicinity, I would sometimes go in to see her off my own bat and I found there was none of the old wear and tear on my patience that I used to suffer. I realized that just being willing to open a door to listen and try to understand had broken through the barrier between us.

This was the year that big changes began in our Wilverton practice.

It was typical of Fred that he was still attending refresher courses like the one at Hollinbourne even though he knew he was heading for retirement. But I think it was the bout of 'flu decided him. Though, typically, he was back in harness in the minimum amount of time, he confessed after a week or two that he was finding night work just too much; besides, he was already old enough to take his pension and retire. So, at the next practice meeting, we reluctantly had to accept his resignation.

We prayed together about a suitable candidate to replace him. 'Better be extra careful this time,' Charles looked in my direction, 'or we might get another like you and then where would we be?'

'Really making progress,' I answered. It isn't good for Charles to get away with things like that.

An old missionary friend of his 'just happened' to let Charles know that his son was near to completing his post-qualification training and that he would soon be looking for a position in general practice.

We liked Francis from the start – cheerful, practical and well-qualified. He'd been married just a year. Soon after he joined us, he suggested a well thought-out rota system for our work, and we adopted it. All things considered, it seemed as if we'd backed a winner in Francis. The outlook for the practice looked bright.

However, as Charles once said, when we were in the middle of a hectic epidemic, 'Life isn't easy in general practice, but it's interesting', and the minor bombshell that burst upon us next was certainly of considerable interest.

Of course, we had known for years that the lease on the St Arkel surgery was running out, but then there was always a written-in option to buy. What we didn't know was that no building society, insurance company or finance house would be willing to lend money on this property. We hadn't realized that the market was so tight.

One agent came round. 'Not viable,' he said, waving a lordly hand at our nice old converted coach-house. 'Suggest you knock it down and start again – we'd lend you money to build a new surgery.'

'And where do you suggest we practice in the meantime?' asked Charles. The agent did not consider this his problem.

There seemed to be no door though this particular 'wall', but all was not lost as it turned out. . .

The Varient engine went thrumming along by the side of the wall – this one was nine feet high and pleasantly red-bricked. As I drove past the opening I saw Mrs Greenaway, head in hands, leaning on the five-barred gate. I waved to her and went on down the little one-way lane which ended in a row of terraced cottages fifty yards on. I was due to see Miss Grant, who lived in the end one, with her widowed sister.

Miss Grant was a courageous old lady who loved gardening. The trouble was that she had severely arthritic knees. Last week I had tried her on a tablet, Butazolidin, which although it had some risks attached to it, could produce remarkable results. It did with Miss Grant. She felt so much better that she had indulged in an absolute orgy of weeding, and now she was laid up with her knees more swollen than ever.

Having duly admonished her and put her on a reduced dose, I went back up the lane. Mrs Greenaway was still at the gate. We were old friends. I stopped the car and got out.

'Hullo, you're looking pensive,' I said.

She looked at me with an air of defeat. 'I've decided to sell up.'

I knew at once what it was all about. Two years before, just as I was beginning surgery, a frantic call had come in. I had raced to that gate in the wall, flung it open and run down through the nursery to find Mr Greenaway face down in the pond at the bottom. I'd hauled him out, but he was dead – drowned in about eighteen inches of water. At the post-mortem the pathologist had found the reason: a blocked brain artery. He had had a stroke and collapsed into the pond.

He and his wife had run a highly successful little business with greenhouses and plots in that beautifully sheltered walled area which had once kept the big house up the hill, now a nursing home, in fruit and vegetables all the year round. Mrs Greenaway had tried to carry on, but she'd obviously now realized it was too much and was finally giving up.

'Oh. I'm so sorry. Can you not get a young chap to help out in the heavy work?' I asked.

'Never make enough to cover his wages,' she answered.

Just then a thought struck me, but I hardly liked to voice it. It sounded so much like cashing in on her misfortune.

'Mrs Greenaway, forgive my mentioning this – but if you are determined to sell up, would you possibly give us first refusal on the purchase of the property? We're looking for new surgery premises at this very moment.'

Her sad face lit up. 'Doctor, I'm so glad! Do you know, I've been thinking for a long time what a wonderful quiet spot this would make for a nursing home or a surgery or something like that? Of course I'll give you first refusal.' Then her face fell. 'Oh, but I was forgetting – I've handed the whole thing over to an agent. You'd have to see him – but of course I could tell him that I want you to have first refusal.'

I was far from impressed when she told me who it was she had engaged. Handle and Friend had a name for slickness. They'd handle her business all right, but I doubted whether anyone would end up still being a friend.

I think Mrs Greenaway must have given them some pretty firm instructions, however. Without too much delay they contacted us and we arranged a pretty fair price. They gave us a written acceptance of our offer, after we had given them a deposit, and all seemed to be plain sailing.

The shop and the house, all built on one storey, would convert amazingly well into a surgery, and the land around seemed tailor-made for use as a parking area for our patient's cars and our own. We would be on our own, quiet and secluded. With potentially such a good set-up, the General Practice Finance Corporation's agent came down to view the property and said they would be only too ready to advance the capital, given a favourable surveyor's report.

Then the delaying tactics began. Every time we contacted the agents there was a new snag. We kept asking for contracts to be exchanged but there was always something holding us up: their solicitor was ill, title deeds had gone astray . . . The weeks slipped by.

Then suddenly it came – their final word. They required the deal to be completed within one week and the money paid over, or it was off.

I knew the score. A little bird (we kept a flock of them among our patients) told us that Messrs Handle and Friend had had a far better offer from a developer. Although we had their written agreement they wanted to get off the hook.

'Can't be done,' our solicitor told us. 'Not in a week.

141

There are searches, title deeds, lots of things – we'd never get a search done in a week.'

'We'll see,' I said.

I needed a search done urgently, I told the clerk at the Town Hall. He happened to be a patient. 'It'll take several days,' he said.

'Look, this is urgent. You want to have a surgery to come to, don't you? Unless you get this for me by tomorrow, you soon won't have one!'

The next day the senior partner of the firm of solicitors rang me up. 'What did you do to the Town Hall?' he said. 'I've got the search by the morning post. Now what about the money?'

It was impossible, of course, to get the GPFC loan in the time, so I went to the bank manager.

'Would you consider lending us £15,000 as a bridging loan for a few weeks?'

He gulped and his eyebrows shot up. He didn't answer for a moment and then he said, 'Well, of course, doctor, as we know you.' He was only speaking the truth – I had prescribed for his gout just the week before. 'I think we can trust you. Now when do you want it?'

'Tomorrow,' I said.

His eyebrows started climbing again. He managed to reply eventually in a voice which suggested someone agreeing to jump blindfold into a pool. 'That will be all right, doctor.'

Next day, to the ill-disguised chagrin of Messrs Handle and Friend, we completed the transaction, paid over our cheque and took possession of our premises.

'Sort of symbolic, that single gate in the wall,' said Charles, as he, Francis and I wandered around our newly-acquired domain later that day. We *had* seemed to be up against a brick wall, until we found an opening.

Elisabeth and I were talking it over in bed that night. 'That American psychiatrist with his door-in-the-wall idea had got something, hadn't he?' I said – though I wasn't thinking of our troubles in the property market just then.

Elisabeth had been very quiet. I wondered if she were asleep – I know my voice does have a soporific effect.

142

'Darling,' she said at last, 'do you know what I'm thinking? I reckon the best illustration of your old barrier wall is in the Bible. You know, where Jesus says, "Look, I'm standing outside the door and knocking. If anyone hears and opens the door, I will come in." We can either leave the barrier there, or open the door and let God into our lives.'

How is it that women so often seem to get it right?